Ketogenic Diet + Intermittent Fasting

Get Results in Half of the Time by Combining Ketogenic Diet + Intermittent Fasting

2 in 1 Special Edition

☐ **Copyright 2017 by Steve Blum - All rights reserved.**

This document is geared towards providing exact and reliable information in regards to the topic and issue covered. The publication is sold with the idea that the publisher is not required to render accounting, officially permitted, or otherwise, qualified services. If advice is necessary, legal or professional, a practiced individual in the profession should be ordered.

- From a Declaration of Principles which was accepted and approved equally by a Committee of the American Bar Association and a Committee of Publishers and Associations.

In no way is it legal to reproduce, duplicate, or transmit any part of this document in either electronic means or in printed format. Recording of this publication is strictly prohibited and any storage of this document is not allowed unless with written permission from the publisher. All rights reserved.

The information provided herein is stated to be truthful and consistent, in that any liability, in terms of inattention or otherwise, by any usage or abuse of any policies, processes, or directions contained within is the solitary and utter responsibility of the recipient reader. Under no circumstances will any legal responsibility or blame be held against the publisher for any reparation, damages, or monetary loss due to the information herein, either directly or indirectly.

Respective authors own all copyrights not held by the publisher.

The information herein is offered for informational purposes solely, and is universal as so. The presentation of the information is without contract or any type of guarantee assurance.

The trademarks that are used are without any consent, and the publication of the trademark is without permission or backing by the trademark owner. All trademarks and brands within this book are for clarifying purposes only and are the owned by the owners themselves, not affiliated with this document.

Contents

Introduction 6
PART I – BACKGROUND INFORMATION 10
Chapter 1. The False Promises of Carbohydrates 11
Chapter 2. The Chemistry of Eating 27
Chapter 3. How We Get Fat and Sickness from Food 37
Chapter 4. Ketosis and Ketogenesis 44
PART II – Ketogenic Diet 54
Chapter 5. Ketogenic Diet Basics 54
Chapter 6. What to Eat. And What Not to! 64
Chapter 7. Do's and Don'ts 76
Chapter 8. Happy Keto Eating Recipes 78
Conclusion 118
REFERENCES 119
Intermittent Fasting 124
Introduction 125
Chapter 1 – What You Need to Know about Fasting 126
Chapter 2 – What Happens to Your Body When You Fast? ... 129
The Benefits of Intermittent Fasting 131
Chapter 3 – The Common Myths about Fasting 134
What are the main perks of engaging in IF? 138
Chapter 4 – The Different Methods of Fasting 140
Chapter 5 – Essential Tips to Make the Diet Work 148
   Chapter 6 – Frequently Asked Questions about Intermittent Fasting 151
Chapter 7 – Foods for Weight Loss 158

Conclusion 167

Introduction

Much has been made of all sorts of quick-weight loss, and fad diets, all delivering the promise of a slimmer figure, glowing good looks, and good health forever and ever. Unfortunately, that is all that they deliver: PROMISES. The slimmer figure and good looks may last for a little while, but the good health facet may not even be achieved even if the weight loss objectives are met.

The problem with these diets is that they were only designed for short-term weight loss, and if we really want to talk about diets, we know that over 97% of dieters get back the pounds that they have lost, and in many cases, actually gain more than what they originally weighed in the first place!

That is for only one diet - people spend a lot of their time going on diets, and the results are hardly successful. In a 2007 study, it was learned that women spend, on the average, 31 years of their lives going on a diet; just exceeding the number of years that men spend, 28.

Another problem with diets is that they usually require a drastic change in the eating patterns. Many require a dramatic drop in caloric intake. Some diets require that people eat tasteless and unappealing foods, making them want to end their diets quickly, and they just revert to their old eating patterns.

The diet that I will lead you through, Ketogenic Diet, is not a fad diet, and its underlying principles have been around for decades. In fact, Ketogenic Diet has not only been a sure-fire approach to weight loss. It has been used to treat certain health conditions, and help others avoid various illnesses.

Our Ketogenic Diet journey will be an educational one on nutrition and diet, and ultimately, a ticket to a better body, and glowing health. This book is divided into two parts, with Part I (Chapters 1 to 4) providing a background on the nutrition and health aspects of any diet. In Chapter 1, we will look at the roles of fat, carbohydrates, and protein in our nutrition, including a history of how humans have regressed to increasing rates of obesity, heart disease, and metabolic problems.

In Chapter 2, we look at how the human body uses the foods that we eat, and convert them into energy and tissue. Chapter 3 describes the body's descent into obesity, including the role of carbohydrates in this sometimes deadly process. We will talk about the various ailments and diseases that arise from a nutrition program with faulty information and premises. In Chapter 4, we review the concept of ketogenesis in detail, including the mechanics of how and why ketones are produced.

Part II of the book (Chapters 5 to 8,) will discuss the how to's for starting on, and progressing with Ketogenic Diet. Chapter 5 will discuss the objectives of the diet, including the significance of ketosis, and provide dieting patterns and schedule to follow. Chapter 6 will detail what foods should be eaten in the diet, and what should be avoided.

Chapter 7 will discuss the basic pointers on how to succeed on the diet. On the flipside, the chapter will also point out what traps to avoid. Chapter 8 gets down to the real world of Ketogenic Diet: Actual recipes that will provide you with a week's worth of meals, snacks, and even desserts, with an emphasis on getting you on a tasty and flavorful track to a healthier life style.

Ketogenic Diet has had a growing number of devotees and fans because of the documented success of millions who have tried it. There are also a growing number of health professionals, including M.D.'s and dieticians who have gone public in promoting the benefits of Ketogenic Diet.

A growing number of nutritionists have also begun to assail the prescribed "balanced" diets that continue to be endorsed by official, national and international medical associations and even, governments. Many Ketogenic Diet devotees now dismiss these official pronouncements as downright wrong, and even, dangerous.

In this book, we will set the record straight on dietary fat and more precisely, its role in the human health and well-being.

We will see that dietary fat deserves to be elevated as THE food nutrient of choice, and should be consumed in at least equal quantities, as carbohydrates and proteins. Fat is not only recommended, but required, as a component of healthy eating and well-being, to help assure you a life of optimal vitality and health!

PART I – BACKGROUND INFORMATION

Chapter 1. The False Promises of Carbohydrates

Mankind's original fuel

All engines need fuel and energy, and human beings, as the most complicated naturally-occurring engine in existence, is no exception. While we put gasoline as fuel in cars, as human beings, we also need to have our own fuel, and this fuel is food. More precisely, food that will be needed in relatively large amounts, consumed consistently and regularly.

Our fuel, food, is comprised of three basic macronutrients: carbohydrates, fat and protein. Everything we eat as fuel for storage and energy comes from these three macronutrients. The human body needs these to function properly. How has the consumption of macronutrients changed over the last 10,000 years or so and what has brought us to this world of dieting and more correctly, failures in dieting?

Gog

Let me introduce you to "Gog," a typical ancestor from our prehistoric days, from about 10,000 years ago, give or take a few hundred years. Gog was a male member of the most advanced and latest version of homo sapien, of which we eventually became the proud descendants. In that stage of human history, Gog was part of that group called the "hunter-gatherers," who sourced their food from animals that they hunted and killed, and from fruits or berries that they happened to come across in their hunting adventures.

Gog and other co-inhabitants of the planet at that time subsisted on a diet that consisted mostly of animal fats, protein, and fibrous berries and fruits. Their Vitamin D source was principally the sun, and they had little use for plant carbohydrates, from whose chlorophyll content merely transfers the sun's Vitamin D nutrients.

Gog stayed out in the sun for most of the day, and the sun provided his "D". Vitamin D was, and continues to be important to sustain the human's bodily functions, but it is clear that fat was to be the human's primary source of fuel.

It is important to note that even today; certain tribes and cultures subsist on essentially high-fat diets and thrive with robust health. The Maasai group in Africa and Eskimos are modern day cultures that are known for the very small part that carbohydrates play in their diet. These groups are sustained by high fat diets in particularly unforgiving weather conditions. Apparently, their low-carbohydrate lifestyles have turned their metabolisms around to fat burners, rather than glucose burners.

This low-carbohydrate situation seemed to be the way that nature designed humans and their fuel needs: Man got their energy from fat, and fat was their fuel. For millions of years, the genius of nature, or even the genius of a Creator deemed that fat would be man's primary source of energy.

Was this simple diet enough for Gog's sustenance and health? For this, we can look at the archaeological record. On the next page, we present a table that shows life expectancy from the year 9,000 B.C., when agriculture, tilling the soil for carbohydrate foods, is generally is known to have started.

TABLE 1.

Life Expectancy of Our "Lithic Ancestors"

Period of Time	Ave. height -male	Ave. height - female	Life expectancy - Male	Life expectancy - Female
30,000 to 9,000 B.C. (Meat and fat is about 2/3 of the diet)	177.1 (5'9.7)	166.5 (5'5.6)	35.4	30.0
9,000 to 7,000 B.C. (Some agriculture already started – Meat and fat is now less than	172.5 (5'7.9)	159.7 (5'2.9)	33.5	31.3

1/3 of the diet)				
7,000 to 5,000 B.C. (Agriculture spreads widely in the Early Neolithic age – Meat is now 30% of the diet)	169.6 (5'6.8)	155.5 (5'1.2)	33.6	29.8
5,000 to 3,000 B.C. ("Late Neolithic," i.e., the transition	161.3 (5'3.5)	154.3 (5'0.7)	33.1	29.2

towards full blown agriculture is mostly complete)				
3,000 to 2,000 B.C. (Early Bronze Era)	166.3 (5'5.4)	152.9 (5'0.2)	33.6	29.4

The above table shows that when humanity began the agricultural stage, life expectancy actually decreased! The decrease should actually have been bigger if we factor in the increased physical security that our ancestors had because of agriculture: enclosed communities and better defensive mechanisms and positions against predatory animals. In fact, deaths from predators on the general population would be reduced to almost zero, with fatalities coming from predators only occurring with the armed male hordes that elected to hunt for animals.

Gog consumed just what his body required, and most of what he consumed was fat from whatever animals he hunted down. The fat he consumed was burned immediately and quickly, not because of physical activity per se, but because the human body, unlike a car, consumes and uses up energy even while he is in a state of rest and even sleep.

From Chapter 2, we will learn that the carbohydrates he consumed were immediately expended for quick bursts of energy. Gog therefore used his nutrients efficiently and effectively, not requiring much fat to be manufactured or stored. This is something we will come back to later in Chapter 4, when we talk about the mechanics of the diet.

"Post" Gog

The archaeological record also shows that as agriculture began to produce more food, agricultural plant products began to play a bigger role in the human diet. When human beings retreated into safer and cozier settlements, there was less of a need to go out and secure animal foods for food. Also note from the table, that males had higher life expectancies than females, even when their lives appeared to be in more mortal danger, being the hunters.

Humans, especially the male hunters, often turned into prey for the animals of the day. Despite this, males still had higher life expectancies because they presumably ate more of the fat that they hunted, possible consuming much of their meat immediately after securing them, and even before distributing them to their waiting families.

In a couple of thousand years more, meat, and especially fat, would continue to take a backseat to processed carbohydrates. Agriculture would become more efficient, and humans would not only produce more of carbohydrate foods, especially in the form of wheat and rice, they could store these foods longer!

For example, wheat and rice could be pounded down to flour, and stored in silos and bins over long periods of time. Because they could be stored longer, they became a much cheaper and more available source of sustenance and nutrition. After all, why risk lives hunting for food when it could be retrieved in a matter of minutes from a storage bin?

<u>Health problems increase</u>

As time marched on, life expectancies would increase as humankind learned more about medicines, while infant mortality rates would plummet. By the Middle Ages, average life expectancies would approach 50 years or so, but other mortal problems would surface: obesity, heart disease, and metabolic issues. Increased carbohydrate intake would totally throw human metabolic processes into crisis.

Before we get into the science and chemistry of food, we can historically trace these problems to one thing: Humans stopped eating naturally, and more importantly, reduced their intake of fat. Millions of years of eating unprocessed foods and fat were in the millennial blink of an eye, overturned, and the human body was shocked, and not pleasantly, to the new nutritional realities. Natural and fat was out, processed and carbohydrates were in. So-called blood diseases, and all sorts of unidentified diseases, presumably cancer and diabetes, began to spread.

Modern Man Doubles Down on the Carbohydrate Problem

From the middle ages to well into the 20th century, humankind saw an increasing, if not alarming incidence of heart disease and symptoms reflecting diabetes. Archaeologists, who have studied heart disease not surprisingly, found that heart disease was extremely rare in pre-industrial societies. After the so-called "Industrial Revolution," which gave witness to large-scale mechanization, heart and metabolic diseases shot up, and people were all of a sudden getting sick in newer ways. Heart attacks and symptoms attributable to strokes suddenly took hold.

Modern conventional wisdom, however, attributed this rise in diseases to the sedentary lifestyle that the advances in technology, especially the invention of machines, brought. The thinking was people were getting fatter and sicker, not because of food, but because people were doing less manual labor than from thousands of years ago. "Experts" assumed that fat deposits formed because people didn't exercise or were sitting, or lying around more.

What they missed or ignored was how human diet was drastically transformed when agriculture took over the human food supply. Modern technology not only made people move around less, it also helped mass produce agricultural products at a faster and cheaper pace.

After wheat and rice were produced in huge, mass proportions, sugar production finally became widespread in the 1700's, and made food, especially, carbohydrates, taste much better. Well into the 1900's, foods high in processed carbohydrate content, such as pizza, French fries, candies, and processed dairy foods gained shot up in popularity.

Moreover, processed carbohydrates became popular because of the short amount of time required to prepare, and with the advent of the microwave oven, cook them. Fast food became a symbol of modern society, and these foods are mostly all about carbohydrates in most of its forms: popcorn, potato chips, and candy bars being the most widespread and popular.

The growth of carbohydrates was largely ignored as a cause of increased heart disease. Because the true villain for human health was being overlooked, a boogeyman had to be found or invented – dietary fat.

Fat gets a bad rap

Sometime in the 1990s, fat was beginning to get demonized. It quickly became the dirty word of the nutrition industry and it was fashionable to shun as a deadly health hazard. Doctors derided it as a scourge to physical well-being, and consumers followed the medical herd, making fat as the primary source of a bunch of physical ailments, most of them revolving around the heart. High "bad" cholesterol, weight gain, artery disease, you name it – all of these were blamed on fat.

The curious thing about the demonization of fat was that there wasn't (and there still isn't) adequate scientific proof to back up these claims of nutritional Armageddon arising from fat.

Despite what science failed to prove, everyone jumped on the low-fat bandwagon, consuming mass quantities of food that, while indeed lacking fat, were instead, loaded with carbohydrates, especially sugar. The results of this "diet revolution" were that the average American got more obese, and the rate of increase of heart problems hastened.

According to U.S. Department of Health and Human Services statistics, by 2001, roughly a third of the American population was already overweight. This, of course, came with the increase in the incidence of heart disease and diabetes also soared.

The result of this "conventional wisdom" was that fresh whole foods such as meat, eggs, and their fatty components—the foods our ancestors ate for centuries—were being quickly replaced with low-fat "Frankenfoods" such as margarine, low-fat snack cookies, and skim milk. These foods were not only full of sugar and carbohydrates; some were also loaded with artificial ingredients. When these substances are consumed regularly, over time, the human body reacts by gaining weight, showing symptoms of fatigue and brain fog, and succumbing to chronic conditions.

Although scientific research produced findings to the contrary, fat—especially saturated fat—had developed a lasting reputation for being bad. Although the low-fat diet craze eventually dwindled, the damage was done. Fat was shunned and carbohydrates were placed on the nutritional pedestal.

In fact, government authorities began to promote, and still promote, the consumption of mostly carbohydrates, for their recommended dietary combinations. The National Institutes of Health, for example, continue to suggest that 70% of a diet should be comprised of carbohydrates in various forms. Subsequently, in the "Dietary Guidelines for America, 2015-2020," issued by the U.S. Department of Agriculture, dietary fats are merely mentioned almost as a footnote as oils.

The USDA also says that food oils (not fat) are limited to fat in liquid form, while naming vegetable cooking oils as the only source of fat nutrients that should be available for human consumption. There is no mention of the animal fat that our ancestors like Gog consumed, which was actually the main source of his energy fuel. The USDA caps their dismissal of fat by allowing very limited consumption levels of animal fat for the "ideal" diet.

To disseminate this fat-starved diet, the USDA pictorialized their concept of an ideal diet with the "My Plate" diagram, which portrays this dismissal of animal fat from the daily diet. The "Plate" emphasizes vegetables, fruits, grains, and protein, and assigns dairy as a supplemental item on the plate diagram. This diagram suggests that at least sixty percent of a person's recommended calorie intake should be comprised of foods from carbohydrates, which make up grains, vegetables, and fruits.

Fats from non-aquatic animals as beef, pork, and lamb, have been excluded in the nutritional conversation, with the "Plate" admonishing everyone to shun the so-called "trans-fat". Government agencies' objective is to limit the consumption of red meat, cheese, and processed meats.

The USDA recommended "Plate" is depicted as follows:

HEALTHY EATING PLATE

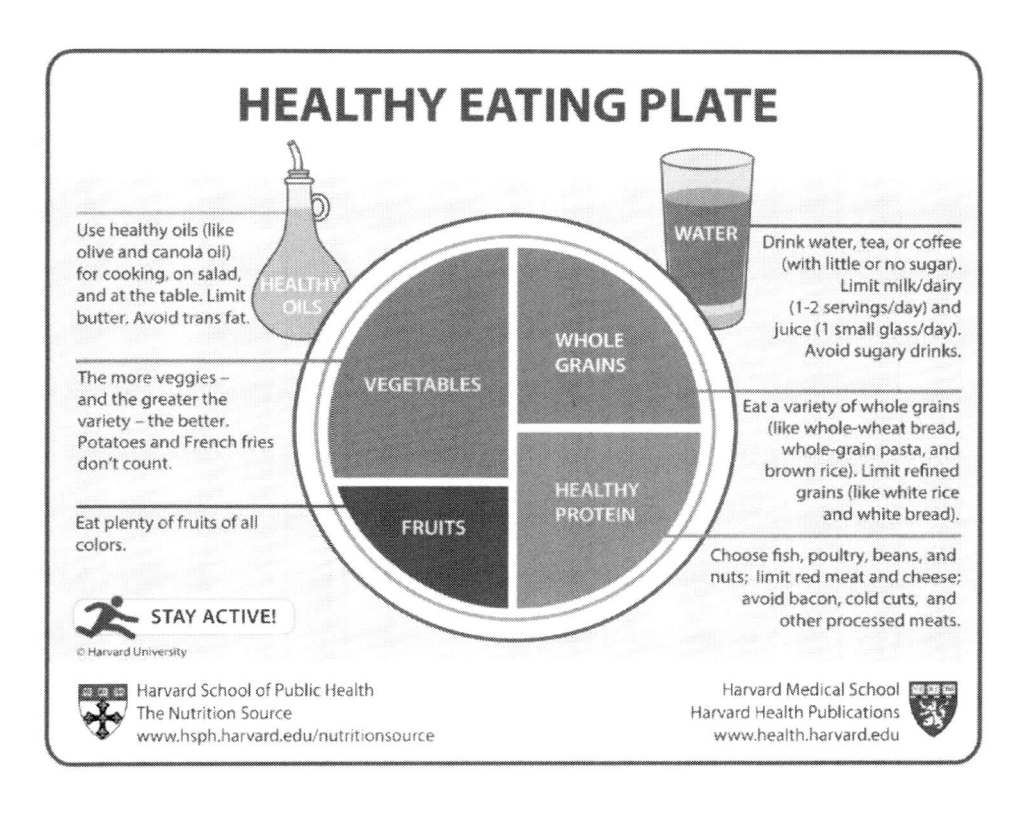

Use healthy oils (like olive and canola oil) for cooking, on salad, and at the table. Limit butter. Avoid trans fat.

The more veggies – and the greater the variety – the better. Potatoes and French fries don't count.

Eat plenty of fruits of all colors.

STAY ACTIVE!

© Harvard University

Drink water, tea, or coffee (with little or no sugar). Limit milk/dairy (1-2 servings/day) and juice (1 small glass/day). Avoid sugary drinks.

Eat a variety of whole grains (like whole-wheat bread, whole-grain pasta, and brown rice). Limit refined grains (like white rice and white bread).

Choose fish, poultry, beans, and nuts; limit red meat and cheese; avoid bacon, cold cuts, and other processed meats.

Harvard School of Public Health
The Nutrition Source
www.hsph.harvard.edu/nutritionsource

Harvard Medical School
Harvard Health Publications
www.health.harvard.edu

Source: U.S. Department of Agriculture

Nevertheless, many current scientific studies have not only repudiated the omission of animal fats from the diet, but have argued that fat from animals is not just a necessary component of the human diet, but should be accepted as the largest part of human nutrition. This is especially true when someone is endeavoring to lose weight, and eventually, get healthier.

The USDA, the National Institutes of Health, the World Health Organization, our grandparents, physicians, and even our gym instructors have been telling us what to eat. Now after we have followed their recommendations, and of course, our own palate, we consume the food and enjoy them. Sometimes, we don't really enjoy these, but just follow the herd to appear to stay modern and in touch. Regardless of what we eat, certain things happen in our body to convert all those goodies into energy.

Chapter 2. The Chemistry of Eating

In Chapter 1, we mentioned that food is the fuel that provides human beings with energy. The three macronutrients, carbohydrates, protein, and of course, fat are the fuels that power our bodies 24/7, day in and day out, whether we are moving around, resting, or even sleeping. In this chapter, we see the role of the macronutrients in the sustenance of our bodies, and how food is converted into fuel and other substances in our body.

Our bodies are highly intelligent, and yet, "needy" machines. They know exactly what they want, and more importantly, what they need. The most unconscious of these needs, and yet probably the most important, is the need for fuel to provide our bodies with energy. Without these energy sources, our cells would starve to death.

You see all these shows and movies about people stranded in islands, forests, and deserts without food? Those are the consequences when your conscious minds and bodies cannot get the fuel necessary to function, and endure.

The first step, the easy and conscious part; chewing and swallowing, puts food into our bodies. The next, more important, however subconscious step; happens inside our body -- to break down this food for absorption, and conversion into energy. This process is called metabolism.

Eating up

Metabolism describes the chemical reactions that take place to maintain the dynamic state of our bodies and their constituent cells. Metabolism has two subordinate bodily functions to process the food/fuel, which we can conveniently divide into the following:

Catabolism – This refers to the breakdown of the molecules that we ingest. The macronutrients are broken down in substances and molecules that can be usable for the body to convert into fuel and energy.

Anabolism - This refers to the amalgamation of all compounds needed by the human body. Basically, in this stage, the body takes what has been broken down by catabolism, and processes the molecules to convert them to energy.

When we ingest the foods that contain the macronutrients of carbohydrates, fat, and proteins, our bodies immediately begin to work on the foods that we take in. The last conscious effort we have in this process is the swallowing of the foods that we have either chewed or drunk. When the mass of chewed food and/or liquids have passed our throat, and heads down our esophagus, the rest of body takes over beyond our conscious control. What happens to these foods?

In order to make sure that it always has access to energy; our body has several metabolic pathways it can use to convert the food that we eat into useable energy, and energy that we can store. We will summarize what these metabolic pathways are all about in the rest of this chapter.

For human beings, the default metabolic pathway is one that uses the glucose from carbohydrates as fuel. As long as you provide your body with carbohydrates, it will use them as energy, and storing excess macronutrients as fat in the process. When you deny your body of carbohydrates, it has to turn somewhere else to get the energy it needs to live. For millions of years up to about 9,000 years ago, the human body turned to mostly, stored and dietary fat.

Anabolism– fed and fasting states

In the metabolic process, a distinction also has to be made between the "fed" and the "fasting" state when the nutrients are being broken down during the anabolic stage. The fed state occurs about 4 hours after eating a meal or snack. This is the time when the body begins to absorb the digested nutrients. Some of these nutrients, especially carbohydrate-based ones, are used to meet immediate energy needs, while converting the extra nutrients to energy stored products.

In the "fasting state," which occurs 4 or more hours after eating, the body uses fat as its main source of energy. How fat or thin we are, depends on how much of fat stores are used, and of course, how those stores are built.

Let us now discuss these blessed little fuel sources.

<u>Carbohydrates</u>

These are probably the tastiest of all foods, the "lightest" on the mouth and the palate, the easiest to swallow, and from an economic standpoint, the cheapest. Rice and wheat for example, can be expanded to 2 or 3 times their original uncooked mass, then laced and mixed with all manner of sugars, creams, flavors, and texturized ingredients to provide the tastiest satisfaction from the lips to the tongue.

After we ingest carbohydrates, these are immediately broken down, by the introduction of various enzymes, into glucose, which is basically blood sugar. Some of the glucose is burned for instant energy, but usually, there is excess glucose left in the blood stream to trigger the body to try to regulate these increases in glucose.

Glucose is the body's favorite source of energy on demand, and is the fuel of choice for athletes, bodybuilders, and gym rats. This is why we have "sugar boosts" after consuming an energy bar or cookie, after a workout or an athletic exercise. The metabolic process that glucose undergoes is called "glycolysis," where the glucose is converted to mostly glycogen.

In the human body's infinite wisdom, it knows that too much glucose can be a problem (which we will see in a while.) To regulate the level of blood sugar, the body lets the pancreas release insulin, a regulating hormone. From this we can see that nature has considered carbohydrates to be inherently bad for the human body, otherwise, why limit it?

Indeed, nature has planted an organ in our body, the pancreas, to produce a singular hormone, insulin, to prevent the body from taking on too much blood sugar. We will visit insulin again in the next chapter when we talk about the effects of sugar and fat on the body.

<u>Proteins</u>

Proteins are responsible for creating the "building blocks" of our body tissues. The most common forms are lean meats and certain legumes. The foods containing protein provide more of a "chewing" sensation before being swallowed, provide the most "filling" sensation, and are more expensive per ounce, than carbohydrates.

Proteins are broken down into amino acids, and used by body cells to form either new proteins or to mixed up in some kind of amino acid "pool". This pool serves like a cache for the molecules, creating some sort of reservoir. Amino acids comprise a significant percentage of our body mass. A big percentage of our cells, tissues, and muscles are also comprised of amino acids.

Amino acids, therefore, perform a bunch of key body functions. One of the most paramount is giving our cells their form and structure. The metabolic process that protein undergoes is called "transamination," where the amino acids we eat are converted to glycogen or other protein compounds.

Aside from forming body tissues, amino acids play an important part in the storage and transport of essential nutrients. They have significant influence over the functions of arteries, glands, organs, and connective tissues, such as tendons. They also are indispensable for repairing tissues, and healing wounds, most especially in the skin, hair, bones, and muscles. Proteins also play an important role in the elimination of various waste deposits arising from metabolism.

Just as ingesting too much of carbohydrates is an issue, the body will need to "dispose" of "extra" amino acids produced over and above the body's requirements. The excess amino acids are transformed by enzymes in the liver into urea and keto acids. These keto acids can then be utilized as extra sources of energy, and via different anabolic processes, are transformed into glucose, or stored in the muscles as fat. Urine and sweat takes care of eliminating urea from the body.

Fat

Fat can be yummy, and can be gross at the same time, but fat is the king of human body fuels; nature having decreed it as the best source of energy. Fat from foods usually is ingested as part of other food items. For example, one can eat the fatty part of steaks, the skin of chickens, and the fat from fish, and egg yolks. Pure fat can be taken in limited forms: of such foods as whole milk and fried eggs.

When fats are eaten, they are converted into fatty acids and glycerol. They are digested in the person's small intestine. They are then turned into lipoproteins for different essential functions (we will talk about bad and good cholesterol, LDL and HDL in the next chapter).

Getting energy from carbohydrates, proteins, and fat

When you eat, the nutrient molecules are absorbed in the intestine and into the bloodstream. In the fasting state, the cells will soon be taking up these nutrients and chemically burn them to liberate energy. The most common chemical fuel is the sugar glucose. Other molecules, such as fats or proteins, can also supply energy, but they usually have to first be converted to glucose or some intermediate that can be used in glucose metabolism.

This is where the energy superstar, adenosine triphosphate, or ATP, comes in. After all the three macronutrients are metabolized, ATP, a critical element in human metabolism, is produced when the body burns the sugars together with other nutrients. Mitochondria in the cells convert the food that we eat into ATP, which is a comparatively smaller molecule which functions as "energy intermediate" when we metabolize food.

ATP is often referred to as "chemical currency" as the body uses it as a direct energy source. The body produces ATP when it burns up various nutrients and sugars, while our cells ingest ATP when engaging in actions such as producing movement, and on an atomic scale, building larger molecules.

Our cells then chemically process ATP, resulting in the release of energy, in order for the human body to engage in various activities.

In essence, our body cells take out the chemical energy from different nutrient molecules such as proteins and carbohydrates, and then utilize this chemical energy to produce ATP. How do we go from glucose to ATP? This is achieved through the process of "oxidation".

For example, glucose, the molecule that came from our consumption of carbohydrates, including many dietary sugars and starch, are broken down to make waste products like water and carbon dioxide. But our cells will utilize the energy freed up from breaking down a single glucose molecule, and produce about thirty ATP molecules.

As soon as a cell has produced ATP, it will now utilize the ATP to meet any of its energy requirements. Cells require energy in order to produce large molecules, such as hormones, for example. Muscle cells also make ATP to generate movement. As a cell produces a large molecule, ATP molecules are broken down. The cell utilizes this energy to produce original bonds among smaller molecules resulting in the production of a bigger one, and the process goes on.

All these processes occur amazingly without our conscious effort or thinking. Our bodies are amazing machines that do all these processes automatically. If we take in the right foods in the right amounts, there shouldn't be any problems. However, since the age of agriculture dawned on humanity 9,000 years ago or so, our bodies have unfortunately, not been so lucky.

Chapter 3. How We Get Fat and Sickness from Food

We now have an idea of how the body processes the macronutrients. Let us pay attention to the negative side of eating, and what happens when we take in too much of the "wrong" types of food into our bodies, especially carbohydrates. In the previous chapter, we mentioned that our bodies were "intelligent" in the singular sense that it tells us when we need fuel, and signals our bodies to take in food whenever our energy sources are getting low.

On the flipside, however, our bodies cannot be "smart enough" to totally withstand bad nutrition, which is eating foods that were not originally designed for our consumption. Despite our bodies' best "efforts," we become obese and sick, and there is very little that it can do from a self-defense standpoint to fight this. In nutrition, the worst thing that can happen to the human body, aside from not being fed enough, is being fed too much, and worse, being fed too much of the wrong foods.

The sugar curse

It may seem that carbohydrates, especially sugars, will be demonized in this, and other books, as the benefits of low-carb, high-fat diets continue to portray as the correct way towards proper weight loss and good health. Actually, as we have seen in the previous chapter, sugar by itself, is not the problem. In fact, we talked about the importance of glucose, and how even proteins and fats are broken down to make sugar in the body.

Glucose is absolutely essential to life, and our metabolism cannot function properly without it. Each cell in our body is able to utilize glucose as energy. Even when we cannot obtain glucose from our diet directly, we can get what we need from fats and proteins. In fact, we have a constant supply of it in our bloodstream. But it can also create severe problems.

Too much sugar

We have discussed how processed carbohydrates, because of their lower price, accessibility, and taste, have become the most consumed macronutrient. The fact that they are also the "lightest" on the mouth and the palate, added to carbohydrates' promotion as the preferred macronutrient, it has practically ensured that human beings will eat them more than any other food.

But sugary and carbohydrate-packed foods are also the most easily converted and metabolized macronutrient. They pass through the digestive tract the fastest, and these factors combined ensure that too much of carbohydrates can be eaten, especially if the habit is picked up when we are young. The bottom line is that anytime we fill our bodies with more than the needed fuel levels, the storage capacity of our liver for sugar is exceeded, and sometimes, greatly.

The liver can store up to only around 5% of its mass as glycogen, which has been converted from excess glucose. When the liver is packed at close to full capacity, the excess sugars are transformed by the liver into more fatty acids.

Worse, these fatty acids go back into the bloodstream, and is distributed throughout our bodies and stored as fat! These fats are stored away where our bodies are designed to store these as adipose fat cells. These areas include, but not limited to, the popular regions of the butt, breasts and hips for women, and the stomach for men. These fatty cells can also imbed themselves in the arteries, causing arteries to deteriorate and being clogged with fat and debris from extra fat.

As a disastrous reverse bonus, as soon as these areas become full with fatty tissues and adipose cells, they will start to leak over into our vital organs – these include the kidneys, liver, and heart. The presence of fat will impair and impede the organ's ability to perform, raise blood pressure, lower metabolic rates, cause a feeling of constant tiredness, and expose the body to illness and sickness as our immune system is weakened.

The body pushes excess glucose into the cells to be made into ATP, or stored as glycogen which are converted into fat droplets called triglycerides in the fat cells, or adipose tissue. "New fat" has just been created.

<u>The wrong sugars</u>

Compounding the "too much" sugar problem is that we may not only be eating too much of carbohydrates, but humans, more than ever, are consuming the wrong carbohydrates. "Gog" and our prehistoric ancestors filled their bellies with natural berries, natural wild fruit, and natural fibers. The operative was natural, and Gog only ate foods that nature provided.

Today, however, there are a vast multitude of foods that contain sugars that nature did not intend us to ingest. Many foods, especially desserts, have sugar (sucrose) and high fructose corn syrup. These are sweetening agents that help enhance the taste of many foods and drinks – practically all non-diet sodas and ice creams contain them.

These are very different from natural sugars that contain glucose, which is an essential life giving nutrient, taken in the right quantities, but fructose is another matter. The molecule is not part of our normal metabolism and we do not produce it. A tiny fraction of cells in the human body can make use of it except liver cells. Since these cannot be properly assimilated into other cellular functions, they get turned to fat, and are eventually secreted into the blood.

Insulin and the Big D- Diabetes

We mentioned in the previous chapter that our bodies are intelligent enough to know that carbohydrates, and especially, processed sugars, are not good for the body, and it takes great pains to try to mitigate the effects of bad dietary habits. One of its best defense mechanisms is the pancreas, which secretes insulin to help mitigate the creation of too much blood sugars and fats, the results of which can be devastating, as we have seen above.

Insulin plays an indispensable role in the body. Its biggest role is its interaction with glucose to let our bodies utilize glucose properly as energy. The pancreas, the organ which produces insulin, excretes enough insulin and it acts as some sort of a "key" that allows the cells of the body to take in, and use glucose as energy.

Insulin assists in controlling blood glucose levels by alerting muscle cells, fat cells, and the liver to extract glucose from the blood. If our bodies have sufficient energy, insulin alerts our liver to process the incoming glucose, and store it as glycogen.

The glucose that insulin "pushes" in to the cells in the form of glycogen can then be transformed into ATP, or stored as fat as described earlier. This additional stored glycogen can then be utilized later on when the body needs more energy. When our bodies experience a disruption in the balance between fat production and the secretion of insulin, diabetes will occur.

Type1 Diabetes

This form of diabetes has also been called insulin-dependent diabetes or juvenile-onset diabetes, and accounts for less than 10 percent of all diabetes cases. Usually a genetic affliction, in this diabetes type, our body's immune system kills the cells that are responsible for releasing insulin, which in effect, stops insulin production.

Type 2 Diabetes

This is the type that Ketogenic Diet will most likely try to address. Type 2 diabetes is the most common form of diabetes (over 90% of diabetes cases), and is usually the result of a diet with very high in carbohydrates. The ones suffering the disease will manifest any symptom prior to diagnosis. Usually Type 2 diabetes is found during adulthood, although a few cases have been known to have been diagnosed in children.

In this affliction, our bodies cannot process insulin the right way. While the most common root cause is still debatable, there is a growing consensus that this is a "lifestyle" disease emanating from an overconsumption of carbohydrates. The bottom line is that the ability of the body to produce insulin has been overwhelmed by the amount of glucose produced. This condition is called, "insulin resistance," and eventually, the body will make less and less insulin, leading some to require insulin injections.

Since Type 2 Diabetes is a lifestyle disease, the way to deal with it is to change our lifestyles! This is best done by going on Ketogenic Diet, and getting the body into the ketosis state.

Chapter 4. Ketosis and Ketogenesis

The human body was designed to use fat for energy, and when mostly fat is used for energy, it does not store that fat, and the body becomes lean, as nature designed it. From Chapter 2, we found out that our bodies have several metabolic pathways it can use to convert the food that we eat into useable energy. The default metabolic pathway is one that uses the glucose from carbohydrates as fuel. As long as you provide your body with carbohydrates, it will use them as energy, storing fat in the process.

When you deny your body with carbohydrates, it has to turn somewhere else to get the energy it needs to live. If you starve your body of carbohydrates, therefore, the body will burn fat, and in the metabolic process, it will produce something called, "ketones." These are what may save your life!

Ketones are organic compounds that are made in the liver from fatty acids, and are generated from the breakdown of fats, especially when the body cannot "locate" any glucose to turn into energy. Ketones are formed almost as a defensive action by the body. When it "senses" that there is not enough sugar or glucose to provide for the body's energy needs, it immediately creates an alternative fuel source.

The Creation of Ketones and Ketosis

During times of fasting, or when we intentionally follow a low-carbohydrate diet, it turns to fat for energy. In simple terms, fat is taken to the liver where it is broken down into glycerol and fatty acids through a process called beta-oxidation. The fatty acid molecules are further broken down through a process called ketogenesis, and a specific ketone body called acetoacetate is formed.

If we continue on Ketogenic Diet, over time, our bodies will adapt to using ketones as fuel, and our muscles will convert the acetoacetate into beta-hydroxybutyrate or BHB. BHB is actually the preferred ketogenic source of energy for your brain, and acetone, most of which is expelled from the body as waste.

When dietary carbohydrates are suddenly taken away from the diet, more fatty acids are released from fat cells, which leads to more fat cells being burned up in our liver. This increase in the burning of fatty acids in the liver eventually causes ketone bodies to be produced, and induces ketosis, a new metabolic state.

Other hormones are likewise affected, and these help transfer the use of this new fuel, instead of carbohydrates, to body tissues. The majority of calories burned up by the human body will now come from this fat breakdown.

The glycerol created during the beta-oxidation process enters into a stage called gluconeogenesis. During gluconeogenesis, the body converts glycerol into glucose that your body can use for energy. Your body can also convert excess protein into glucose. Your body does need some glucose to function, but it doesn't need carbohydrates to get it. In other words, during this period, our body is beginning to now burn fat instead of converted sugar! Ketosis has set in, and hopefully for good!

So is fat and ketosis bad?
Ketogenic Diet has been at the forefront of a big diet "revolution" for the past few decades. Its popularity continues to increase, as new scientific evidence continues to surface, and proves that fat does not deserve the bad nutritional reputation it has received. Is fat bad?

The human body was designed to use fat for energy, no matter where it is produced. This results in a lean body, as nature originally designed it. How does a dieter on Ketogenic Diet get to ketosis? Getting to a state of ketosis means ingesting less than 50 grams of carbohydrates per day, and in the next Chapters we will find out how to count these carbohydrates, including the tools you need to measure carbohydrate intake.

Weight loss in Ketogenic Diet

Now that you understand how your body creates energy and how ketones are formed, you may be still wondering just how this translates into weight loss. Let's provide a quick review and summary.

When you eat a lot of carbohydrates, your body happily burns them for energy and stores any excess as glycogen in your liver, or as triglycerides in your fat cells. When we take carbohydrates out of the equation or reduce our intake of them drastically, our body depletes its glycogen stores in the liver and muscles and then turns to fat for energy.

When our bodies start to burn stored fat, our fat cells shrink and you begin to lose weight and become leaner. Smaller, leaner cells = smaller, leaner bodies!

Ketosis has sometimes been confused with ketoacidosis, which is a pre-existing condition present in some diabetic patients. It is a condition where there is not enough insulin produced in the body. Ketosis is not ketoacidosis, and vice-versa. Ketosis will not lead to ketoacidosis, and assuming you have no other medical conditions that may prevent you from going on Ketogenic Diet.

While many people try to dismiss Ketogenic Diet as a dangerous fad diet, it is well worth noting that the diet has many helpful, life-changing, and life-saving effects on our bodies and long-term health. Weight loss and looking great is sometimes viewed as merely side benefits by those who have stayed on the diet for an extended period of time.

There are other ways on how Ketogenic Diet can contribute to your well-being and long life. If you understand what amazing benefits are in store, it will be very easy to get convinced to stay on the diet. Described below are the foremost benefits of going on Ketogenic Diet.

Elimination of Type-II diabetes

We mentioned that Type-II diabetes is a lifestyle issue, and that it can be cured by a lifestyle change. For diabetes, the best lifestyle change is to get on Ketogenic Diet, and stop letting carbohydrates ruin your health. Many Type-II diabetes conditions are treatable before requiring the use of injected insulin.

Reduction of the symptoms of epilepsy

Ketogenic Diet is sometimes recommended to help control seizure symptoms in some patients afflicted with epilepsy. Ketogenic Diet is prescribed by a doctor and the patient undergoes careful monitoring under the watch of a professional dietitian.

Reduction in the symptoms of cancer

Cancer cells are very much not like our healthy cells. One way that they have known to be way different is that they have about ten times as many more insulin receptors on their surface as ordinary cells. The receptors allow the cells to feed on nutrients and glucose coming from the bloodstream at a very significant rate.

The more carbohydrates that are catabolized, the more glucose are produced which helps the cancer cells gorge for their "nutrition." If we are able to remove carbohydrates from our diets, we can possibly deny cancer cells from their energy source.

Reducing the incidence and severity of Parkinson's disease and Alzheimer's

Parkinson's disease is one of those "motor system" disorders where the onset happens between the ages of 50 and 65 years old. In the United States, about 1 percent of people in that age group are affected with it. In Parkinson's disease, the dopamine-producing cells in the brain are seemingly destroyed. The symptoms of Parkinson's disease include slowness of movement, trouble with balance, tremors, and shaking.

Near the terminal phase, the victim is usually on a wheelchair, or bed-ridden. These symptoms show up after up to 80 percent of the dopamine-producing cells in the brain are devastated. While it is not exactly clear on how Ketogenic Diet can alleviate the symptoms of Parkinson's disease, it is highly possible that ketones, which have an anti-inflammatory effect on the brain, may be able to fix impaired neurons.

The ketones may also possibly bypass the area in the brain that is damaged, and bring much-needed energy to other areas in the brain.

Reduction of symptoms of Mitochondrial Disorders

Mitochondria are organelles that are of significant numbers in most human cells. This is where the essential biochemical processes of energy production and respiration take place. Mitochondria are also considered as the energy centers of the human body. They convert the food that we eat to adenosine triphosphate, or ATP, as we have learned in Chapter 2.

When mitochondria become dysfunctional, the cells are denied of the energy they need. Because the brain, muscles, heart, nervous system, and eyes demand the most energy, their cells are often the most significantly affected with a mitochondrial disorder. Affecting these body parts cause learning and intellectual disabilities, muscle weakness, hearing and visual impairment, respiratory disorders, and even seizures. There is no cure for mitochondrial disorders, so their treatment focuses on alleviating its symptoms and improving the quality of life of the sufferer.

Proper diet is often the first stage of therapy for these disorders, and with seizures are a common symptom, a high-fat, Ketogenic Diet is often part of the treatment plan.

Reduction of symptoms of Lou Gehrig's or ALS Disease

ALS (Amyotrophic Lateral Sclerosis) is a progressive, neuro-degenerative ailment that assaults the nerve cells in the spinal cord and brain. ALS specifically affects the motor neurons, which are responsible for voluntary muscle movement. When motor neurons die, they are no longer able to send nerve signals to the muscle fibers leading to slurred speech, difficulty swallowing, muscle weakness, and almost instantly fatal breathing. At any rate, most of the muscles begin to waste away, and the person affected becomes weaker.

The exact cause of ALS is unknown, and there is no cure for the disease. Researchers believe that disruptions of the mitochondria in the brain and changes in a person's diet may help those with ALS, as well. Studies on mice and other animals show that those under Ketogenic Diet experienced a greater decrease in symptoms than those who weren't.

Improved Focus and Mental Clarity

For the brain, exposure to too much glucose can result in neurotoxicity or the exposure of the nervous system to toxic substances. Many mental issues, such as brain fog and problems with memory, are caused by this condition. In Ketogenic Diet, the reduction of the supply of glucose diminishes the levels of toxicity in the body as brain starts to use ketones as fuel. Possible results are the ability to think more clearly, better focus, and better memory recall.

Increased Energy

When the body breaks down fat instead of carbohydrates, more energy is produced for each ounce of fat used, leaving the Ketogenic dieter with a feeling of heightened alertness and increased energy.

Better heart and coronary health

When there are less fat cells flowing through the blood stream, that means that there is less strain on the heart and the arteries. This is a result of less plaque clogging up the bloodstream, and a better functioning circulatory system.

Lower "bad cholesterol" levels

Weight and fat loss are the objectives of an overwhelming majority of people going on Ketogenic Diet. Of course, the associated benefits of a slimmer body can also lead to a decrease in "bad" cholesterol levels, blood pressure, and just better heart health.

Breaking the myths surrounding high fat diets

It is useful to know what people, even health professionals, can say to scare people from Ketogenic Diet. There are many myths and misconceptions that have surrounded, and clouded ketosis and Ketogenic Diet.

Ketosis myths

Myth 1: Carbohydrates are an essential nutrient for good health.

Myth2: Eating a low-carbohydrate diet can lead to vitamin deficiencies, especially Vitamin C, which come from carbohydrate-rich sugary fruits and vegetables.

Myth 3: Ketogenic Diet causes your body to go into ketoacidosis, which is dangerous.

Myth 4: Your kidneys will sustain damage from high fat consumption.

Myth 5: A high-fat diet will lead to osteoporosis, because it will cause the body to excrete calcium.

Myth 6: Eating fat makes you fat.

Myth 7: Ketogenic Diet leaves out carbohydrates completely.

Myth 8: Cholesterol from animal fat causes heart diseases.

PART II – Ketogenic Diet

Chapter 5. Ketogenic Diet Basics

Before we get into the nitty-gritty of the diet, an important few words on how Ketogenic Diet is different from other low-carbohydrate diets on the market.

Atkins Diet

Atkins Diet was at the forefront of the low carbohydrate revolution and brought ketosis and ketogenesis into public awareness about fifty years ago. Atkins Diet allows for a moderate amount of protein in the menu. The allowable ratio is about 50-35-15 in terms of fat/protein/carbohydrate ratio. In Ketogenic Diet, the overwhelming amount of calories should come from fat, about 70%.

Atkins Diet also puts a lot of emphasis on the two week, "induction" phase, where the dieter will have to consume the required macronutrients. Atkins Diet promoters claim that a person can lose up to fifteen pounds on the first week of the diet.

Atkins Diet also allows the dieter to slowly reintroduce certain carbohydrates after the induction period. On Ketogenic Diet, the dieters need to be on a high fat diet for the rest of their lives.

Paleolithic Diet

Paleolithic Diet focuses on the foods supposedly eaten by our prehistoric ancestors, just like Ketogenic Diet, and also reduces the emphasis on carbohydrates. But Paleolithic Diet also allows for more significant portions of vegetables and certain fruits. Certain grains are allowed, and in fact recommended. Like Ketogenic Diet, Paleolithic Diet forbids tubers and sweet potatoes. The big difference between both diets is that high fat dairy products can be consumed on Ketogenic Diet, but is expressly disallowed on Paleolithic Diet.

Other diets that promote lower carbohydrate intake

Two other famous diets, Zone Diet and South Beach Diet, also recommend carbohydrate intake significantly lower than that of Ketogenic Diet. However, they allow for the consumption of a wider variety of carbohydrates. Ultimately, only Ketogenic Diet dictates that the significant majority of macronutrients consumed should be from fat.

The importance of macronutrients

Our body's overwhelming source of fuel is the food that we eat. Some of our energy comes from sunlight (Vitamin D), but 99% of our fuel comes from macronutrients in the food that we eat. Ketogenic Diet's effectiveness depends almost wholly on what we eat and drink. There is no need for supplementation, such as vitamins when we go on Ketogenic Diet.

Think of the macronutrients as the gasoline that we put in our cars. Taking in the wrong macronutrients can be compared with putting contaminated fuel in your gas tank, or putting diesel fuel, for example, in a car that requires high-octane gasoline.

In Ketogenic Diet, the proper fuel is fat.

Getting on Ketogenic Diet

a. Prepare your household and cupboard for Ketogenic Diet

Going on a high-fat diet means a big change in lifestyle. If we are not living alone, and have to share our cupboards, refrigerators, and shopping budgets with other people, we need to properly announce that things will be changing drastically in the food storage department.

On Ketogenic Diet, carbohydrates are the big enemy, and we have to make sure that no "stealth carbs" manage to intrude our food space. Be organized, create lists, and shop carefully. We go into much greater detail on what we need to eat in the next chapter.

b. How many grams of protein, carbs and fats should be eaten in Ketogenic Diet?

In Chapter 1, we mentioned that most "authorities" recommend that about two thirds of calories should come from carbohydrates. This means that for a typical daily diet of 2,000 calories consumed, at least 1,300 calories of the total should be consumed in the form of carbohydrates. Additionally, around 500 calories should come from protein, and the remainder, should come from incidental, and trace quantities of fat.

Remember that these so called authorities do not even contemplate fat as being a food group, but only gives some token credit to fats as oils added to foods for taste and use in food preparation.

Ketogenic Diet turns this all around. Dietary fat should now make up about two-thirds of daily calorie consumption, allowing a maximum of ten percent to come from carbohydrates. Converting this to food weights, this means that under Ketogenic Diet, we should only consume daily between 30 and 50 grams of carbohydrates.

The more active a person is, however, a little more carbohydrates are added, maybe up to 100 grams, can be eaten. This is a concession to the fact that carbohydrates are useful for those that require short-term bursts of energy, such as those who go to a gym or exercise regularly and athletes.

For protein, the recommended quantity can be between 115 grams and 175 grams per day. The rest of the diet should be concentrated on fat. For a 2,000 calorie daily diet, we need to ingest at least 60%, or 1,200 calories of fat, 25%, or 500 calories from protein, and 15%, or 300 calories, from carbohydrates.

A note on protein which we have given very little attention to: Proteins are important in the creation, maintenance, and repair of muscle tissues. We want protein to rebuild our tissue, and not be an inefficient source of energy. In fact, excess proteins can turn into fat, the way carbohydrates are converted.

c. Recording and monitoring calorie and macronutrient intake

To ensure of the success of the diet, we need to carefully monitor how much of each macronutrient we are consuming daily, to ensure that the right proportion of calories are being consumed.

There are a multitude of carbohydrate/calorie counters that are available. The preeminent source is the suite of Atkins Diet publications that pioneered the high-fat revolution. These need to be purchased in publication or app form.

A good source to look for apps is http://www.mydreamshape.com/carb-counter-apps/

Regardless of whether you record your progress in a written journal, or monitor yourself via computer, tablet, or phone, you need to strictly be in compliance with the percentages I have just mentioned. This monitoring is especially important in the first few weeks, when you are transitioning your body into the ketosis state.

Of course, you need to pay strict attention to the actual macronutrients you can (and should not!) consume when you are on the diet.

d. Signs That You Are in Ketosis

Signs that you're in ketosis may start appearing after only one week of following a true Ketogenic Diet. For some people, it can take longer—as much as three months. The amount of time it takes for you to start seeing signs that your body is burning fat for fuel largely depend on you as an individual. When signs do start to show, they are pretty similar across the board.

"Keto Flu"

"Keto flu" or "low-carb flu" commonly affects people in the first few days of starting Ketogenic Diet. Of course, Ketogenic Diet doesn't actually cause the flu, but the phenomenon is given the term because its symptoms closely resemble that of the flu. It would be more accurate to refer to this stage as a carbohydrate withdrawal, because that's really what it is.

When you take carbohydrates away, it causes altered hormonal states and electrolyte imbalances that are responsible for the associated symptoms. The basic symptoms include headache, nausea, upset stomach, sleepiness, fatigue, abdominal cramps, diarrhea, and lack of mental clarity, or what is commonly referred to as "brain fog."

Carbohydrate addiction is a real thing. Some research shows that carbohydrates activate certain stimuli in the brain that can be dependence-forming and cause addiction. Carbohydrate addicts have uncontrollable cravings for carbohydrates, and when they do eat them, they tend to binge. For a carbohydrate addict, the removal of carbohydrates can cause withdrawal symptoms, such as dizziness, irritability, and intense cravings.

The duration of the symptoms varies—it depends on you as an individual, but typically "keto flu" lasts anywhere from a couple of days to a week. In rare cases, it can last up to two weeks. Some of the symptoms of the "keto flu" are associated with dehydration, because in the beginning stages of ketosis you lose a lot of water weight.

With that lost fluid, you also lose electrolytes. You can replenish these electrolytes by drinking enhanced waters (but make sure they are not sweetened) and drinking lots of homemade bone broth. This may help lessen the severity of the symptoms.

Bad Breath

Unfortunately, bad breath is another early sign that you're in ketosis. When you're in ketosis, your body creates acetone as a waste product. Some of this acetone is released in your breath, giving it a fruity or ammonia-like quality. You can combat bad breath by chewing on fresh mint leaves and drinking plenty of water, since bad breath is also associated with dehydration.

Decreased Appetite and Nausea

As your body adapts to Ketogenic Diet, you may have a decreased appetite. This is because you're providing your body with plenty of fat and protein, which are both highly satiating, and not a lot of carbohydrates. The nausea associated with "keto flu" can also decrease your appetite. When you reach this stage, it's important that you eat even if you feel like you aren't hungry. You want to make sure your body is getting enough calories and nutrients, especially in this time of transition.

Increased Energy

When the fog begins to clear and your body starts to become keto-adapted, the uncomfortable symptoms you were feeling will dissipate and you'll begin to see the benefits of following Ketogenic Diet. One of the first beneficial signs many people experience is an increase in energy. When your body breaks down fat instead of carbohydrates, more energy is produced gram for gram, leaving you feeling alert and energized.

Other Possible Signs

Cold hands and feet

Increased urinary frequency

Difficulty sleeping

Metallic taste in the mouth

Dry mouth

Increased thirst

Chapter 6. What to Eat. And What Not to!

Shopping for the right foods is the first and most important step short of putting the right food in the mouth. For today's food shopper, fortunately, most food manufacturers are sensitive to the needs and requirements of people who go on special diets such as Ketogenic Diet. In labeling their foods, they have endeavored to be more accurate and responsive to people who need the proper information to go on their diets.

Regardless of whether foods are "allowed," the serious dieter will still have to make sure that they are staying well within the required macronutrient ratios (preferably 65% fat, 20% protein, and 15% carbohydrates). If measuring ratios are not possible during a given meal, the overriding principle is that the majority of the calories eaten daily should come from fat, and a very small percentage should be from carbohydrates.

Quality

The "quality" of your food matters, especially when it comes to fat and protein sources. Going back to the prehistoric time, our ancestors got healthy on unprocessed and unrefined food alone. It would be healthy and beneficial if a diet plan replicates that prehistoric food profile. A Ketogenic dieter should also try to purchase foods that have the following descriptions on the labels: organic, grass-fed, free-range, and/or pasture-raised.

Food with labels that say, "farm-raised" should be avoided as much as possible, because in all probability, whatever has been "raised" in those "farms" have been sprinkled with a healthy dose of chemicals and preservatives to improve yield and increase the animals' sizes.

Meats, poultry, and seafood

These are the staples of Ketogenic Diet, not vegetables, rice, or grains. They are the most plentiful, and in fact, appetizing components of the diet, and contains naturally-occurring fat. There are many foods in this group that most people can eat all they want every day. Foods included in this food group comprise all types of beef, chicken, turkey, duck, fish, lamb, pork, shrimp, crab, and lobster.

Of course, "exotic" varieties such as ostrich, goat, deer, and buffalo, are also allowed, if available. While bacon and sausage are excellent sources of protein and fat, care should be taken in eating processed meats, especially hotdogs and sausages. Many brands contain substantial quantities of carbohydrate fillers.

Remember that when eating meat, make sure to stay within your recommended protein grams for the day, since your body converts excess protein into glucose via glucogenesis, which can kick you out of the ketosis state.

In the following lists, we will show what the carbohydrate and fat contents are for a particular food item. Remember that these measurements are for uncooked and undressed food. Because Ketogenic Diet is ultimately a low-carbohydrate diet, we are listing the carbohydrate content of each food item. We will also list the number of calories for each item. Note that there may be many varieties of food types, especially in the meat items, because meat comes from various parts of the animal.

The list below is a fairly large general representation of foods that we generally eat. In the reference section of this book, I provide some resources for carbohydrate and calorie counting, in general.

a. Foods that are good for Ketogenic Diet

      Animal Meats:

Beef/Veal – 3 oz. has 0 carbohydrates, and about 300 calories

Pork - 3 oz. has 0 carbohydrates, and about 200 calories

Lamb - 3 oz. has 0 carbohydrates, and about 175 calories

Goat - 3 oz. has 0 carbohydrates, and about 100 calories

Venison -3 oz. has 0 carbohydrates, and about 150 calories

Other wild game:

Keep in mind, the organic and grass-fed meat. Even if they are a little more expensive, they are the healthiest options, because there is a much lesser chance that they will contain growth hormones and preservatives. Game meat has generally less calories than regular pork and beef, and for the most part, has zero carbohydrates.

Processed meats:

While being basically comprised of the same meats that we have just listed that have zero carbohydrates, the curing and processing required to give them taste, sometimes necessitates the adding of carbohydrates.

Bacon – 3 oz. has less than 2 grams of carbohydrates, and about 450 calories

Bologna – 12-gram slice has about 1 gram of carbohydrates, and about 50 calories

Pork rinds - 3 oz. has 0 carbohydrates, and about 300 calories

Salami - 12-gram slice has about 1 gram of carbohydrates, and about 50 calories

Sausage (e.g., Bratwurst, Kielbasa, etc.) - 3 oz. has 2 grams of carbohydrates, and about 300 calories

Make sure that these yummy meats do not contain added sugars or excess preservatives.

Poultry:

You can be liberal with the skin and the fat portions. There is no need to skim them off anymore. Once again, organic and grass-fed cuts are the healthiest options. These include:

Chicken – 100 grams has 0 carbohydrates, and about 120 calories

Duck - 100 grams has 0 carbohydrates, and about 130 calories

Goose - 100 grams has 0 carbohydrates, and about 160 calories

Ostrich - 100 grams has 0 carbohydrates, and about 110 calories

Pigeon -100 grams has 0 carbohydrates, and about 200 calories

Quail - 100 grams has 0 carbohydrates, and about 150 calories

Turkey - 100 grams has 0 carbohydrates, and about 125 calories

Speaking of poultry, eggs, especially the yolk part, are highly recommended. Organic eggs or eggs from grass-fed chickens are preferred.

    Fish – fatty varieties, especially:

Bass - 100 g has 0 carbohydrates, and about 150 calories

Halibut - 100 g has 0 carbohydrates, and about 110 calories

Mackerel - 100 g has 0 carbohydrates, and about 200 calories

Salmon - 100 g has 0 carbohydrates, and about 140 calories

Tuna - 100 g has 0 carbohydrates, and about 150 calories

Trout - 100 g has 0 carbohydrates, and about 150 calories

    Peanut Butter – Check the labels to ensure that the variety is very low in carbohydrates, and have no sugar content. 2 tbsps. of such varieties have about 5 g of carbohydrates, and 200 calories.

    Dairy:

Butter – 0 carbohydrates and 500 calories per 100 grams

Cheese – Make sure that you watch out for blends! They may have sugars and other dangerous chemicals and preservatives to make them look, and taste like real cheese. Most well-prepared cheese without any fillers 100 g has 1.5 g carbs, and about 400 calories

    Plant products:

Asparagus, green – 1 cup has 5 g of carbohydrates and calories

Avocados - 1 cup has 20 g of carbohydrates and 300 calories

Bamboo shoots - 1 cup has 8 g of carbohydrates and 40 calories

Broccoli - 1 cup has 6 g of carbohydrates and 30 calories

Celery stalks - 1 cup has 4 g of carbohydrates and 15 calories

Coconuts – 1 cup has 12 g of carbohydrates and 300 calories

Green, leafy vegetables, such as bok choy, lettuce, Swiss card, radicchio, endives. These are non-starchy vegetables and typically 1 cup has about 5-10 g of carbohydrates and between 25-50 calories.

Kale - 1 cup has 5 g of carbohydrates and 30 calories

Kohlrabi - 1 cup has 8 g of carbohydrates and 40 calories

Radish - 1 cup has 2 g of carbohydrates and 15 calories

Broth, especially self-made bone broth, non-sweet pickles, kimchee, sauerkraut, and mustard.

Almost all herbs and spices (no sweeteners and preservatives) and recipe enhancers such as lime juice, lemon, and their grated skins.

Whey protein - keep away from those with sugar, chemical additives, and soy additives

Nuts (make sure there are no sugar-based additives) such as Brazil nuts, hazelnuts, pecans, walnuts, sunflower seeds, sesame and pumpkin seeds, pistachios, pine nuts, and peanuts.

Oils such as coconut oil, pure lard, and olive oil

b. Take the following in moderation

These can be eaten after the initial phase of ketosis has been completed.

Plants:

Bell peppers, shallots, tomatoes - 1 cup has between 10-20 g of carbohydrates and 30-50 calories

Berry varieties, including strawberries, blackberries, cranberries, raspberries, and blueberries. Berries are tricky because while they have an abundance of sugars, they are rich in fiber, which greatly reduces their "net" carbs, or carbohydrates discounted by the fiber they contain.

Cabbage, cauliflower, broccoli, fennel, rutabaga, turnips, Brussels sprouts, and eggplant

Eggplant - 1 cup has 5 g of carbohydrates and 20 calories

Garlic -1 teaspoon has 1 g of carbohydrates and 4 calories

Leeks – The bulbs and lower leaf portions - 1 cup has 15 g of carbohydrates and 50 calories

Mushrooms - 1 cup has 2 g of carbohydrates and 15 calories

Olives - 1 cup has 5 g of carbohydrates and 20 calories

Rhubarb - 1 cup has 5 g of carbohydrates and 20 calories

Onion - 1 cup has 10 g of carbohydrates and 40 calories

Other Peppers- 1 cup has 10 g of carbohydrates and 40 calories

c. Foods that should be avoided at all costs

Alcohol in most forms. Most pure rums and some vodkas though, have zero carbohydrates. Bar beverages and alcohol-based drinks usually have a lot of sugars and syrups and should be avoided.

However, dieters can also consume a variety of beverages in moderation, as long as they contain no sugar. Check the labels carefully on so-called diet sodas to make sure that they do not contain any sugar. Unlimited drinks will include tea, coffee, and heavy cream, minus any refined sugars or sweeteners.

As with most diet plans, water is still the best bet as a beverage alternative. It is a good idea to drink at least half of your body weight in ounces. Plain water can be infused with fresh herbs, such as mint or basil, to provide a little variety. Sodas, flavored waters, sweetened teas, sweetened lemonade, and fruit juices should be avoided.

High-fructose corn-syrup is that deadly stealth sweetener found in most soft drinks, and juices. We mentioned fructose briefly in Chapter 2. If the "high" in high-fructose is not enough to scare someone away, consider that it also functions like a preservative, meaning that not only does it lack B vitamins and other important nutrients, it is chock-full of chemicals that have no business being in the human body.

Avoid grains and sugars in all of their forms. Grains include wheat, barley, rice, rye, sorghum, and anything made from these products. This means that Ketogenic Diet will have no breads, pasta, crackers, and rice. Sugar and anything that contains sugar is also not allowed. This includes white sugar, brown sugar, honey, maple syrup, corn syrup, and brown rice syrup.

There are many names for sugar on the ingredient lists. It's extremely beneficial to familiarize yourself with these names so you will know when a product contains sugar in any form. Be careful of artificial sweeteners like Splenda that could actually be made out of sucralose, which contains carbohydrates.

Breads, including wheat bread

Breakfast cereals

Chocolate bars and candies

Desserts, especially cakes, pies, and pastries

Energy bars, including protein bars

Energy boost drinks - look for sugarless varieties though

Ice cream

Oils that are processed are generally harmful to the body, and will impede Ketogenic progress. These include margarine, sunflower, cottonseed, safflower, canola, grape seed, soybean, and corn oils.

Pancakes and waffles

Rice

Sodas and sugary drinks, including most juice drinks

Syrups and chocolate toppings

T.V. dinners

The basic rule is this: You have to avoid foods and drinks with sugars, carbohydrates, and chemicals.

Chapter 7. Do's and Don'ts

While Ketogenic Diet can provide some awesome benefits, there are many pitfalls to avoid if one is to have success, and even avoid serious hazards to your health.

Mistakes on going on Ketogenic Diet

Because Ketogenic Diet is a radical departure from what most people are used to, it is easy to make mistakes. The following are the most common mistakes that can remove the benefits of Ketogenic Diet, and may even cause harm to your body:

1. To gain the maximum benefits from the diet, you have to be in a state of ketosis for at least two weeks. You CANNOT deviate from this, or you will basically need to start from zero again.

2. Eating too much processed fats and proteins. This is especially true for boxed or T.V. dinners. While they may have a lot of fat content, there are usually a lot of hidden sugars, and worse, artificial chemicals that can derail your progress.

3. Eating more protein as opposed to fat. Fat is the main source of energy, and eating excess protein is bad, because some of it is converted to sugar.

4. Being afraid of fat. In the dietary world, fat is a friend, and we need to forget all the misconceptions about it.

5. Not getting enough water. Sometimes we drink water to accompany carbs, especially sweets, so drastically reducing carbs may cause us to consume less water. Water is the most important element of any diet, and it sometimes helps to give the body a feeling of "fullness."

Chapter 8. Happy Keto Eating Recipes

<u>Meal Plan for Ketogenic Diet</u>

Congratulations! You've gone this far, and now it's time to be rewarded for your persistence and attentiveness.

This chapter will present 7 days' worth of Ketogenic-friendly meals and snacks, which will contain the bare minimum of carbohydrates, while maximizing the consumption of fats and fatty foods. Eating a combination of the meals will guarantee that you will consume less than 50 grams of carbohydrates per day, and should provide a pretty clear picture of the direction that needs to be taken in order to be successful on the diet. Ketogenic Diet requires this proportion in order for the body to achieve ketosis quickly and consistently.

Breakfast Recipes:

1. Ketogenic Breakfast Muffins

Fat Ingredients:

1 medium Egg

1/4 cup Heavy Cream

1 slice cooked Bacon (Cured, Pan-Fried, Cooked)

1 oz. Cheddar Cheese

Other Ingredients:

Salt & Black Pepper (to taste)

How to Prepare:

1. Preheat oven to 350 F.

2. In a bowl, whisk the eggs with the cream and salt and pepper.

3. Spread into pam sprayed muffin tins, and fill the cups 1/2 full.

4. Place 1 slice of crumbled bacon to each muffin and then 1/2 oz. cheese on top of each muffin.

5. Bake for about 15-20 minutes or until slightly browned.

6. Add another 1/2 oz. of cheese onto each muffin and broil until cheese is slightly browned. Enjoy!

2. Ultra Ketogenic Style Egg Breakfast (Serves 2)

Fat Ingredients:

6 organic eggs

½ cup of heavy cream

1 tablespoon of butter

Other Ingredients:

1 cup of shredded spinach

A small pinch Sea Salt+ ground white pepper

1 small onion finely minced

How to Prepare:

1. Take a mixing bowl. Add the eggs, cream, salt and pepper and beat well and put aside.

2. Take a large skillet and heat 1 tablespoon of butter.

3. Then add the onion and spinach and stir constantly.

4. Next, pour the egg mixture and stir until everything becomes scrambled and cooked till light, fluffy and yellow.

5. Serve hot.

3. Bacon & olive omelet (Serves 4)

Fat Ingredients:

8 large free-range eggs

16 thin slices bacon

Other Ingredients:

20 pitted black olives

Pinch of pink Himalayan or sea salt

Freshly ground black pepper

How to Prepare:

1. Cut the olives into thin slices.

2. Lay the bacon, preferably free-range or organic, equally on the surface of the pan and roast for about 5 minutes.

3. Put the eggs into a mixing bowl with a pinch of salt and pepper and beat them well with a whisk or fork.

4. Turn the bacon on the other side when it gets slightly golden in color.

5. Lower the heat and pour in the eggs equally all over the pan.

6. Use a spatula to bring in the omelet from the sides towards the center for the first 30 seconds.

7. Sprinkle with sliced olives and cook for another minute or until the top appears to be almost cooked and firm.

8. Ease the omelet's edges with a spatula. Turn off the heat and serve the omelet on to a plate.

4. Keto Scrambled Eggs (Serves 4)

Fat Ingredients:

8 large eggs

1 tablespoon butter

1 cup shredded Cheddar cheese

½ cup diced sugar-free turkey or chicken ham

¼ cup heavy cream

Other Ingredients:

1 teaspoon salt

½ teaspoon black pepper

½ cup chopped onion

⅓ cup chopped red and green peppers

Chopped scallions for garnish (optional)

How to Prepare:

1. In a large mixing bowl, whisk eggs, cream, salt, and black pepper.

2. Melt the butter in a medium skillet over medium heat. Add egg mixture and stir.

3. When the eggs begin to scramble, add the ham, onion, and peppers.

4. Continue to stir until eggs are almost cooked. Add the cheddar cheese and stir.

5. Flourless Cream Cheese Pancakes (Serves 4)

Fat Ingredients:

4 eggs

4 oz. cream cheese

Other Ingredients:

1 tbsp. cinnamon

2 tbsp. coconut flour

1 packet of Stevia in the Raw

How to Prepare:

1. Combine/mix all the ingredients in a mixing bowl until smooth.

2. Heat up a non-stick pan or skillet on medium high, and coat it with butter or coconut oil.

3. Pour the batter as if it was a regular pancake batter.

4. Cook on one side most of the way before flipping.

5. Top with butter, and/or sugar-free syrup.

6. Keto Eggs Benedict (Serves 4)

Fat Ingredients:

8 large eggs

2 tablespoon butter

8 slices sugar-free Canadian bacon

2 cups Hollandaise Sauce

1 large avocado, cut into 8 pieces

How to Prepare:

1. Heat up a medium skillet over medium-high heat and add the butter. Crack eggs into the pan. Cook for 2 minutes and then flip eggs, using care not to break yolks.

2. Cook for another 2 minutes or until white is completely cooked, but yolk is still runny.

3. Transfer eggs to a plate.

4. Top each egg with a slice of Canadian bacon and a slice of avocado. Pour the sauce onto each egg.

7. High-Fat Ham, Cheese, and Egg Casserole (Serves 6)

Fat Ingredients:

12 large eggs

2 cups cooked diced cooked ham (make sure this does not contain any sugar)

1/2 cup shredded mozzarella cheese

1/2 cup shredded Cheddar cheese

Other Ingredients:

4 cups broccoli florets

1/2 cup chopped scallions

Bunches of broccoli (approximately one cup)

How to Prepare:

1. Preheat oven to 375°F.

2. Fill a large pot with water and bring to a boil. Blanch broccoli by putting in boiling water for 2–3 minutes.

3. Put eggs, ham, mozzarella, cheddar, and scallions in a large bowl and whisk until combined. Add broccoli.

4. Pour into a 9" × 13" baking pan and put in the oven to cook.

Lunch Recipes

1. Stuffed Avocados (Serves 4)

Fat Ingredients:

2 (6-ounce) cans tuna in oil

4 tablespoons mayonnaise

2 large avocados

Other Ingredients:

1 medium green bell pepper, chopped

1 teaspoon dried minced onion

1 teaspoon garlic salt

1 teaspoon black pepper

How to Prepare:

1. Cut avocado in half lengthwise and remove the pit. Set aside.

2. Put tuna, mayonnaise, bell pepper, dried onion, garlic, salt, and black pepper in a medium mixing bowl and mash together with a fork until combined.

3. Scoop half of the mixture into each half of the avocado.

2. Pork Tacos (Serves: 4)

Fat Ingredients:

25 oz. pork mince

½ cup of goat cheese

½ cup of mayonnaise

Other Ingredients:

3 teaspoons Taco Seasoning

4 Romaine Lettuce Leaves

How to Prepare:

1. Place the pork mince in a skillet and cook it for 20 minutes until nice and brown. Leave to cool.

2. Place the pork mince on the lettuce leaves.

3. Add the seasoning, goat cheese and a dollop of mayonnaise.

4. Wrap securely.

3. Chicken Kebabs (Serves up to 5)

Fat Ingredients:

1.5 lbs. chicken tenderloins (approx. 10)

1/2 tbsp. rosemary olive oil (or regular)

Other Ingredients:

10 6" rosemary skewers (soaked in water for at least 1 hour)

A few sprigs of fresh thyme

1/2 tbsp. garlic salt

1/2 tbsp. lemon pepper seasoning

How to Prepare:

1. Preheat oven to 350 degrees.

2. Soak the rosemary skewers for at least 1 hour in water.

3. Use a short sharp knife to twiddle a point on the end of each stick.

4. Toss chicken with ingredients. Slide the leaves off the thyme sprigs and sprinkle them in.

5. Skewer the tenderloin with a rosemary stick.

6. Bake at 350 F for 40 minutes.

4. Sausage Balls (Serves 10 – good to store)

Fat Ingredients:

2 cups of sausages shredded

½ cup of cheddar cheese

½ cup of cottage cheese

1 egg

1 tablespoon butter

Other Ingredients:

1 teaspoon of chili flakes

½ cup of red peppers

¼ teaspoon of mustard powder

How to Prepare:

1. Preheat an oven to 350 degrees.

2. Add the egg, chili, and red peppers in a bowl and mix/whisk until the ingredients are mixed completely.

3. Mix in the remaining ingredients.

4. Using a wooden baking spoon, or cookie scoop, remove the mixture, and hand-roll the sausage into about two dozen sausage balls.

5. Place the formed balls on a buttered baking pan, or cookie sheet.

6. Bake for about 15 minutes. Serve.

7. You may also store the cooked sausage bags in a covered bowl, or sandwich bags in the refrigerator for later use.

5, Tarragon Tuna (Serves 2)

Fat Ingredients:

Two 6-ounce tuna steaks, 1 inch thick

2 teaspoons mayonnaise

1 teaspoon olive oil

Other Ingredients:

2 tablespoons minced fresh or 2 teaspoons dried tarragon plus tarragon sprigs for garnish

Salt and cracked pepper to taste

How to Prepare:

1. Stir together the mayo and tarragon in a small bowl. Cover and set aside.

2. Heat a heavy skillet or ridged grill pan over medium-high heat.

3. Pat the tuna dry with paper towels, then season to taste with salt and cracked pepper. Dab olive oil over the surfaces of the fish.

4. Pan grilled the fish for about 3 minutes per side for medium. Transfer to warmed dinner plates.

5. Top each steak with a dollop of tarragon mayonnaise, and garnish with tarragon sprigs. Place a mound of squash beside the tuna.

6. Tuna and Egg Salad (Serves 2)

Fat Ingredients:

2 large hard-boiled eggs

2 (6-ounce) cans tuna (try to get those packed in oil

½ cup mayonnaise

Other Ingredients:

¼ cup diced white onion

¼ cup sugar-free relish

½ teaspoon salt

½ teaspoon black pepper

How to Prepare:

1. Put eggs in a medium mixing bowl and mash with a fork. Add tuna and mayonnaise and mash together until ingredients are combined.

2. Stir in onion, relish, salt, and pepper.

7. Chicken Avocado Salad (Serves 2)

Fat Ingredients:

1 (12.5-ounce) can shredded chicken breast

1/2 cup Homemade Mayonnaise

1 teaspoon olive oil

1 medium avocado, cubed

Other Ingredients:

2 tablespoons sliced black olives

1/2 teaspoon garlic salt

1/2 teaspoon black pepper

1/4 teaspoon paprika

1 teaspoon fresh lemon juice

How to Prepare:

Put all ingredients in a medium mixing bowl and mash with a fork until combined.

Dinner Recipes

1. Carb-less Pork Skewers (Serves 4)

Fat Ingredients:

2 lbs. pork shoulder

1 cup virgin olive oil (may be reused later on)

Other ingredients:

Juice from 2 large lemons

2 tbsp. balsamic vinegar

4 tbsp. freshly chopped mint

4 tbsp. freshly chopped oregano

2 tsp. sea salt

Dash of freshly ground black pepper

4 wooden or stainless steel skewers

How to Prepare:

1. To prepare the marinade, rinse the mint and oregano and drain thoroughly. Chop the herbs and preserve these apart in a small bowl.

2. Cube the pork into big cubes. Place them in a medium bowl and pour the olive oil on them.

3. Add the chopped herbs and season with balsamic vinegar. Season with salt and freshly grounded black pepper to taste.

4. Combine all the ingredients, and ensure the meat is submerged in oil. Let it relax in the fridge for 8 to 12 hours.

5. When the meat is marinated, use the grill to preheat the oven to 450 degrees. Note that the meat will barely change color after you take it out from the fridge. This is fine.

6. Skewer the meat pieces in four skewer sticks. Place them on a rack and within the oven.

7. After about 10 minutes, flip the skewers, and cook until done.

2. Sea Bass with Mango Chutney, Ginger, and Black Sesame Seeds (Makes 2 servings)

Fat Ingredients:

Two 6-ounce striped bass fillets

1 tablespoon sesame oil

Cooking spray

Other Ingredients:

1 tablespoon minced fresh ginger (see note)

1 tablespoon soy sauce

Salt and freshly milled black pepper to taste

¼ cup mango chutney

3 cups shredded iceberg lettuce

Ginger and Hot Red Pepper Vinaigrette

How to Prepare:

1. Preheat the oven to 425°F. Spray an 8 X 8 X 8-inch Pyrex baking dish with cooking spray.

2. Place the fillets in the baking dish. Sprinkle each fillet with ginger, soy sauce, and sesame oil. Lightly salt and pepper. Cover the dish with foil and bake for 10 minutes.

3. Remove from the oven and spoon 2 tablespoons of chutney onto each fillet. Return to the oven and bake, uncovered, for 5 more minutes.

4. Toss the shredded lettuce with the dressing. Divide between two plates and top each one with a fillet.

3. Roasted Butterfish (Serves 4)

Fat Ingredients:

Four giant butterfish fillets

8 tablespoon butter or ghee

Other Ingredients:

4 cloves garlic

4 teaspoons freshly chopped thyme

Pinch sea salt

Juice from 1 lemon

How to Prepare:

1. Begin by seasoning the butterfish fillets with a little bit of salt and place them on a plate.

2. Soften the butter, add the herbs and crushed garlic and blend all the pieces collectively in a small bowl.

3. Pour the butter combination over the fish.

4. Warm a non-stick pan over medium heat and add the fish.

5. Roast for about 2 to 3 minutes on both sides until cooked and the fish will get a crispy golden texture. Be certain that the fillet is totally cooked by slicing into it. Cooked flesh will look opaque.

6. Place the fish onto a serving plate and squeeze a little bit of lemon over it. Serve sizzling.

4. Broccoli and Ham Quiche (Serves 12)

Fat Ingredients:

10 large organic eggs or 12 medium eggs

2 cups of thinly sliced ham

1 cup of grated cheddar cheese

1 ½ cups of heavy cream

3 tablespoons of olive oil

Other Ingredients:

12 cups of cubed broccoli flowerets

2 teaspoons of chili flakes

How to Prepare:

1. Preheat the oven to 350F.

2. Take 2 deep 10-inch quiche pans. Grease them with a bit of olive oil and keep aside.

3. Take a large mixing bowl. Crack all the eggs and pour into the bowl. Then add the heavy cream, chili flakes, and beat well until it has all been mixed well.

4. Take each quiche pan and place the ham slices and broccoli flowerets evenly in each pan. Then sprinkle the cheese over them and finally pour the egg and cream mixture over it.

5. Bake for 20 minutes until the top is golden brown in color. Prick with a fork till the bottom of quiche to check if done. If it is clean, then the quiche is ready to enjoy.

5. Baked Salmon (Serves 4)

Fat Ingredients:

4 6-ounce salmon fillets

3 tbsp. olive oil

Other Ingredients:

2 tablespoons of lemon juice

1 tablespoon each of minced parsley, mint, garlic, paprika, sunflower seeds (slightly crushed)

How to Prepare:

1. Clean the fillet and put aside.

2. Place all the other ingredients in another bowl, and mix well and pour onto the fish. Marinate the fillet for 6 hours.

3. After 6 hours, place in a baking dish and bake for 1 hour at 250F until flaky and cooked.

4. Serve with sour cream, green beans and apricots.

6. Fried Chicken (Serves 4)

Fat Ingredients:

1 pound or 4 (4-ounce) boneless, skinless chicken breasts

1/2 cup crushed pork rinds

1/2 cup grated Parmesan cheese

2 large eggs

2 tablespoons coconut oil

Other Ingredients:

1/2 teaspoon garlic powder

1/4 teaspoon onion powder

1/4 teaspoon dried minced onion

1/4 teaspoon salt

1/4 teaspoon black pepper

How to Prepare:

1. Put pork rinds, Parmesan cheese, garlic powder, onion powder, minced onion, salt, and black pepper in a large mixing bowl and stir until well mixed.

2. Crack eggs into a separate bowl and whisk.

3. Dip each chicken breast into eggs and then coat in pork rind mixture, making sure the chicken is completely covered.

4. Heat coconut oil in a skillet over medium-high heat. Place the chicken breasts into the pan. Let them cook for 5–7 minutes or until pork rind crust is browned. Flip chicken over and let them cook for another 5–7 minutes until cooked through.

5. Serve hot.

7. One Pan Baked Chicken Thighs (Serves 2)

Fat Ingredients:

4 chicken thighs (deboned, skin on)

1/4 cup olive oil

Other Ingredients:

2 zucchinis

1/2 cup carrot (sliced)

2 tablespoons balsamic vinegar

1 cup daikon radish

1-inch length of cube ginger, minced

How to Prepare:

1. Pre-heat an oven to 350 degrees.

2. Use a paper towel, and pat the chicken thighs dry.

3. Wrap the skins around the chicken thighs, and place these on a buttered or greased baking sheet.

4. Slice the radish and zucchinis, and with the carrots, place them around the thigh pieces.

5. Using a small bowl mix the vinegar, oil, and ginger – this is your sauce. Pour the mix over the chicken.

5. Season with salt and pepper and bake the chicken thighs for 30 minutes.

Conclusion

I hope this book was able to help you to achieve not only your weight loss goals, but to have a more vibrant, healthier lifestyle beyond losing weight and looking great.

The next step in your journey is to start listing down your weight goals, changing your food shopping lists, and prepare for a new and sexier wardrobe!

Finally, if you enjoyed this book, then I'd like to ask you for a favor, would you be kind enough to leave a review for this book on Amazon? It'd be greatly appreciated!

Thank you and good luck!

REFERENCES

Introduction

1. Brown, H. (2015). Planning to Go on a Diet? One Word of Advice: Don't. Retrieved December 30, 2016, from http://www.slate.com/articles/health_and_science/medical_examiner/2015/03/diets_do_not_work_the_thin_evidence_that_losing_weight_makes_you_healthier.html

2. Average woman spends 31 years on a diet, researchers say. (2007). Retrieved December 30, 2016, from http://www.dailymail.co.uk/health/article-430913/Average-woman-spends-31-years-diet-researchers-say.html

Chapter 1. The False Promises of Carbohydrates

1. Office of Dietary Supplements - Daily Values (DVs). (n.d.). Retrieved December 18, 2016, from https://ods.od.nih.gov/HealthInformation/dailyvalues.aspx
2. USDA "Plate"

2. Choose MyPlate. (n.d.). Retrieved December 25, 2016, from https://www.choosemyplate.gov/

3. Longevity/Health in Ancient Paleolithic vs Neolithic Peoples. (n.d.). Retrieved December 20, 2016, from http://www.beyondveg.com/nicholson-w/angel-1984/angel-1984-1a.shtml

4. DeWitte, S. N., & Bekvalac, J. (2010). Oral Health and Frailty in the Medieval English Cemetery of St. Mary Graces. Retrieved December 22, 2016, from https://www.ncbi.nlm.nih.gov/pmc/articles/PMC3094918/

5. A Brief History of Heart Disease. (n.d.). Retrieved December 22, 2016, from http://forum.prisonplanet.com/index.php?topic=206436.0

Chapter 2. The Chemistry of Eating

1. McDonald, L., & McDonald, L. (1998). The ketogenic diet: a complete guide for the dieter and practitioner. Austin, TX: The Author.

2. Metabolic processes (2010). Retrieved December 26, 2016, from https://www.youtube.com/watch?v=mtHDjC1emGs

3. Overview Metabolism. (n.d.). Retrieved December 24, 2016, from http://chemistry.elmhurst.edu/vchembook/600glycolysis.html

Chapter 3. How We Get Fat and Sick from Food

1. Cordain, L. (2011). The Paleo diet: lose weight and get healthy by eating the foods you were designed to eat. Hoboken, NJ: Wiley.

Chapter 4. Ketosis and Ketogenesis

1. Boyers, Lindsay (2015). The everything guide to the ketogenic diet: a step-by-step guide to the ultimate fat-burning diet plan! Avon, MA: Adams Media.

2. Ray, N. (2013). Atkins diet: complete Atkins diet guide to losing weight and feeling amazing! North Charleston, SC: Createspace.

Chapter 5. Ketogenic Diet Basics

1. Excellent carb-counting resource include:

http://www.carb-counter.net/

2. There are a great multitude of apps for both Android and IOS. Listed below is a tiny sample of what's available:

Calorie, Carb & Fat Counter by Virtuagym

Calorie Counter by My Fitness Pal

Low Carb Foods Guide by deluxapps

3. Boyers, Lindsay (2015). The everything guide to the ketogenic diet: a step-by-step guide to the ultimate fat-burning diet plan! Avon, MA: Adams Media.

4. (2016). Retrieved December 26, 2016, from https://www.youtube.com/watch?v=H7mjm9LyW-c

Chapter 6. What to Eat. And What Not to!

1. H. (2016). Complete Keto Diet Food List: What to Eat and Avoid | The KetoDiet Blog. Retrieved December 24, 2016, from http://ketodietapp.com/Blog/post/2015/01/03/Keto-Diet-Food-List-What-to-Eat-and-Avoid

2, Johnson, R. A., Says, R., Says, J. R., Says, C., Says, L., Says, L., . . . Says, A. (2016). The Ultimate Ketogenic Diet Food List (What to Eat on The Keto Diet). Retrieved December 22, 2016, from https://dietingwell.com/ketogenic-diet-food-list/

3. H. (2016). Ketogenic Diet Food List - What Are Keto Foods? (PDF Download). Retrieved December 20, 2016, from http://paleomagazine.com/ketogenic-diet-food-list

Chapter 7. Do's and Don't's

1. H. (2016). How to Low Carb: 15 Common Weight Loss Mistakes | The KetoDiet Blog. Retrieved December 27, 2016, from http://ketodietapp.com/Blog/post/2016/01/11/how-to-low-carb-15-common-weight-loss-mistakes

2. 13 common keto mistakes. (2016). Retrieved December 22, 2016, from https://www.ketovangelist.com/13-common-keto-mistakes/

Chapter 8. Happy Keto Eating Recipes

1. Slajerova, M. (2016). Sweet & savory fat bombs: 100 delicious treats for fat fasts, ketogenic, paleo, and low-carb diets. Beverly, MA: Fair Winds.

2. The Best Keto Recipes. (n.d.). Retrieved December 23, 2016, from https://www.dietdoctor.com/low-carb/recipes/best-keto-recipes

3. Low Carb Recipes for Ketogenic Diets. (n.d.). Retrieved December 27, 2016, from http://www.ketogenic-diet-resource.com/low-carb-recipes.html

Intermittent Fasting

How to Gain More Muscle, Optimize Fat Loss, and Achieve a Super-Human Focus

Introduction

I want to thank you and congratulate you for purchasing the book, "Intermittent Fasting: Learning about its benefits for diet, weight loss and overall health".

This book aims to inspire you to adopt this kind of diet for weight loss and the other health benefits that it entails.

This book features chapters dedicated to some of the most frequently-asked questions about fasting. You will also learn about several myths regarding it, as it's only by uncovering the truth that you become capable of making an informed decision.

Chapter 1 – What You Need to Know about Fasting

Did you know that humans can survive without food for more than three weeks? Fasting means that you won't eat for a period of time. Intermittent fasting means that you will practice this at irregular intervals. There are different kinds of intermittent fasting, also referred to as IF, which vary with the period of intervals or the covered hours of your eating window.

IF is an umbrella term used to refer to the different kinds of diet programs that have a cycle that comes in between a fasting period to an eating period. Fasting is not a new concept. Fasting is considered a religious practice by many, including those that follow Christianity, Islam, and Buddhism. Fasting is an ancient practice that offers many health benefits aside from weight loss.

Many people who are trying to lose weight have one question regarding IF though – when will you eat? The idea here is similar to falling from the top of an eight-story building. Falling straight to the ground will definitely kill you, but if you fall with someone catching you at each floor, the result is going to be different. The total distance of the fall may be the same, but the impact is not.

The concept of falling from a building is similar to the foods that you eat – they will boost the levels of your insulin to varying degrees. In order to sustain your health and prevent insulin resistance, you have to keep the levels of your insulin low. When you fast, it heals your body and helps you lose weight at the same time.

Do not mistake fasting for starvation. These are two different concepts because with the latter, you are involuntarily deprived of food. The matter is out of your hands – it's something that you can't control, unlike with fasting.

You may not be aware, but you actually do fasting every day. This was how the term, breakfast, came about. It is the meal that is intended to break the fast that you voluntarily subject yourself to while you sleep.

Where did the idea of fasting originate?
It was said that Hippocrates, the father of modern medicine, prescribed fasting to his patients. The reason was summarized to what he has written, "To eat when you are sick, is to feed your illness." There were other known people in ancient history that supported the practice of fasting, such as Plato and Aristotle, and the Greek historian and writer, Plutarch, who believed that it is better to fast than take medicines. The founder of toxicology, Philip Paracelsus, also supported fasting and wrote that the process is the greatest remedy. The idea was supported by one of the founding fathers of America, Benjamin Franklin, who wrote that fasting is one of the best medicines, along with resting.

Many ancient Greeks observed nature and patterned their medical treatments based on their findings. They believed that people have a thing called "the physician within". They don't eat when they are sick. People (and even animals) act instinctively when they are not feeling well. These ancient Greeks also concluded that fasting helps in boosting a person's cognitive skills.

Have you ever binged on food? How did it make you feel afterwards? After having a feast and getting yourself quite full, do you feel good and energetic, or is it the other way around? More people will likely feel tired and sleepy after eating too much. This comes as a result of how your system reacted to getting too much food. When this happens, more blood is pushed to your digestive system and only a little of the blood goes up to your brain. This is actually dangerous and can even lead to food coma.

Fasting is also associated with religious practices, although it may be called by different names (such as purification and cleansing).

It was a shared belief of Buddha, Muhammed, and Jesus Christ that the practice has healing powers.

Fast Facts about the Process

The 2014 review that was done by Valter Longo and Mark Mattson, and was published in the journal, Cell Metabolism, revealed that fasting helped in improving the conditions of the animal models used in the tests. These conditions include sensitivity to insulin, high blood pressure, and inflammation.

According to studies, any kind of diet that involves fasting has to be done along with a plant-based or calorie-restricted diet, in order to gain more health benefits from the process. One of these studies was done by the head of the National Institute on Aging's neuroscience laboratory, Mark Mattson in 2003. He concluded that a calorie-restricted diet resulted to lower levels of glucose and insulin in the blood (do note though, that he conducted the study on mice).

Scientists have been studying the link between reduced calorie intake and fasting as far back as the 1930s. Through time, a lot of evidences emerged, pointing out that reducing calorie consumption by up to 40 percent can extend a person's lifespan. Eating less, especially as you age, can reduce your risk of developing common health problems.

Before you undergo any kind of IF diet though, make sure that you are monitored by a physician, especially if you intend to fast for more than a day. There may be changes in your circadian rhythm and gastrointestinal system that need to be checked to ensure your safety and health.

The IF diet dictates when you should eat and not what you ought to eat. It is more of an eating pattern and it is still up to you what kinds of food you will have during the period.

Chapter 2 – What Happens to Your Body When You Fast?

When you perform fasting, the hormones in your body naturally adjust to the process. As a result, you will experience the following:

1. A boost in growth hormone secretion
This hormone in your system is responsible in increasing the availability of fats that the body can use as fuel. It also aids in preserving the density of your bones, as well as your muscle mass. A common problem that people experience as they age is the decreased secretion of this hormone. This problem is addressed through fasting, which acts as a potent stimulus to hormone production. The secretion of growth hormone can actually double after five days of fasting.

2. More energy
How does that happen? How can you have more energy when you are not eating? Your adrenaline increases as your body experiences an increase in metabolic rate. The added energy is needed to find food, and to get more food after the fast is over. During the process, the body transitions to burning fat instead of sugar for energy. In effect, you are feeding your system with your own fat or the food that it was able to store when you were not fasting or during the hours that you are allowed to eat.

3. Sustained health
You need not worry about malnutrition even if you have chosen to follow a fasting method that will take longer than the other kinds. The fat stores in your body are enough to sustain your health. It is possible for the levels of your potassium to go down a bit, but it will still remain on safe and healthy levels even if you continuously fast for two months. The levels of other nutrients in your body, such as calcium, magnesium, and phosphorous will remain stable. Besides, you can take a multivitamin supplement to meet your recommended allowance of micronutrients daily.

4. Decreased levels of insulin
Since all foods cause a rise in your insulin levels, it only goes to say that avoiding food will cause the opposite effect. Your body will then burn fat, which will maintain the normal levels of the glucose in your blood. This effect can already be felt after a day or two of fasting, but if you want to see a dramatic reduction in your insulin levels, then you would have to do longer-duration fasts.

The Benefits of Intermittent Fasting

Given the growing popularity of intermittent fasting, a lot of people are discovering its benefits. As it continues to be known in many parts of the world, it is also beginning to attract some doubters. The fact is, this kind of diet will only work if you will do it along with the right diet and proper exercise. The diet can make you feel better about yourself, so you will live better and longer.

Here are the other benefits of the IF diet:

- Lower levels of LDL cholesterol and triglycerides
- Lower risks of oxidative stress, problems in your DNA and lipid
- Decreased chances to develop cancer
- Lower blood pressure
- Boosts your system's fat-burning capacity
- Release of growth hormone at the latter part of the fast
- Improved cellular repair and turnover
- Better blood sugar control
- Better function of your cardiovascular system
- Improved appetite control
- Protection against neurotoxins

IF affects your hormones and cells. Once you begin with the diet, the fat stored in your body becomes more accessible. Your cells will automatically undergo repair processes and you will:

1. Experience changes in your gene expression, which will give you protection against a lot of diseases and therefore, will make you live longer.

2. Have improved insulin sensitivity, which will lead to lower insulin levels. This is why fat stores become easier to access and address.

3. Undergo repair processes by removing the old and damaged proteins that have been stored in your cells.

4. Enjoy increased muscle gain and accelerated fat loss (mainly due to the greater availability of growth hormones).

IF is beneficial to your overall health and it also improves your brain function. As you continue with IF, your mental capacity will get a boost as the hormone BDNF in your brain increases, as proven by the 2011 study about dietary restriction, done by Mattson, Duan, Guo and Lee. This hormone aids in the growth of new nerve cells. It helps the brain to function better. It also gives you protection against Alzheimer's disease. This is the reason why many people are raving how the diet can lengthen one's lifespan.

These are only some of the changes that you will experience as you fast. You have to be prepared for more, especially if this is your first time to do it. You might find it hard at first and you might not have the energy to continue doing the normal things that you do. Instead of giving up without giving it a try, this should challenge you to move forward and expect greater changes. You have to think that these changes will later lead to weight loss and improved health.

IF Helps You Lose Weight
Among its many benefits, more people are getting interested in the diet because of its capability to help you lose weight. It leads to the automatic reduction of your calorie intake since you will be having fewer meals. Weight loss is facilitated as the diet changes your hormonal levels. Your system will release the hormone that is called norepinephrine, which is responsible in burning your fats. Even when you resort to fasting for a short period of time, your metabolic rate will increase up to 14 percent. The claim was fortified in a 2015 study by Verpeut, Gotthardt, Yang, Yeomans, Bello, Roepke, and Yasrebi.

You can only imagine what more benefits can you gain when you stick with the diet for a longer duration. You only have to get used to it. Try its different variations until you find the one that will work for you. The kind of diet that you ought to follow will depend on your lifestyle. If you are often involved in physical activities that are tiring and challenging, you cannot suppress your system from food for a long time. It needs to feed on something in order to function well.

Weight loss happens as you take in fewer calories since you are eating less. As a result, your system will burn more calories than how much you are taking in. Studies have shown that IF can actually lead to about 8 percent of weight loss for 3 up to 24 weeks, which is already a big deal when compared to other kinds of diet programs.

Among the body fats that you will lose, around 7 percent will come from your waist circumference. It means that you will lose a significant amount of fat around the belly and the organs that surround it, which will result to decreased chances of developing related diseases. You will also have fewer muscle loss, unlike the other kinds of diet that require restriction in your calorie intake.

It is important to take note that you might likely binge on foods with high-caloric content during the periods that you are allowed to eat. This comes as a result of suppression, especially if you used to indulge a lot in these foods. If you will allow this to happen, you will only regain the weight that you have already lost and your body might find it harder to lose more weight.

You are what you eat and what you do. Fasting will not work on its own. You have to be dedicated and be certain that you remain disciplined all throughout. This kind of attitude is important not only with IF, but with any kind of diet techniques. The success and failure of your diet depend a lot on your attitude. For now, you have to learn as much as you can about the diet. This way, you will know how to counter the side effects and know what to do when cravings strike.

Chapter 3 – The Common Myths about Fasting

No matter what you do, many people will try to dissuade you and tell you about the myths that they have accepted as infallible truths. Here are the most common myths that certain cynics of the diet believe as truths:

1. Eating frequently, even in small portions, can reduce hunger.
There are people who believe that having frequent snacks will take your mind away from food and your cravings. While this may be true for certain individuals, there are studies that proved otherwise. Actually, the results of different studies are mixed. There are some which hinted that it can cause reduced hunger, but there are also studies which proved that it can boost one's hunger levels. It was concluded that it really varies among individuals. You cannot accept the myth as truth without trying first what will and won't work for you.

There are those whose hunger levels are best reduced by having three meals that are rich in protein than six smaller meals of the same kind.

2. You will get fat when you continually skip breakfast.
It has always been said that breakfast is the most important meal of the day. This is why many people perceive that there is something special about it that you would miss out on when you are fasting. The myth is that skipping this meal often could lead to excessive hunger and boost your cravings, which will eventually lead to weight gain.

A study done in 2014 by the researchers at the University of Alabama debunked the myth. After 16 weeks of observing more than 200 obese and overweight adults who were grouped into two (those who eat breakfast and those who don't), it was found that this factor isn't that important to weight loss. Similar to the first myth, whether or not skipping breakfast will help you lose weight also depends on individual characteristics.

3. The brain will not function well without a good supply of glucose.
There are people who aren't keen on the idea of cutting out carbs from their diet. This is based on the fact that the brain uses glucose as fuel. You have to understand that the body is a work of genius. It will make its own glucose if it lacks the supply. This is done through the process of gluconeogenesis. This is rarely needed because the body has stored glycogen in your liver. This is used to give your brain its needed fuel for several hours.

When you fast for a long period and you take in only a little amount of carbs throughout the duration, your system will burn fat and turn them into ketone that will provide the needed fuel for your brain.

Take note though that there are certain individuals who feel hypoglycemic when they fast. If you are part of this group, you have to eat small portions of meals several times throughout the day. It is also important that you seek your doctor's advice before changing anything with your diet.

4. Snacking is good for your health.
Eating often or snacking can actually increase your risk for certain diseases. This is especially true when you snack on foods rich in calories. This can lead to a boost in your liver fat, which will raise your risk of fatty liver problems. There are also studies, which proved that eating often will make you more at risk of colorectal cancer than those who stick to regular meals or the ones who fast from time to time. These studies include the recent one published in the Nature journal. It was headed by Omer Yilmaz, an assistant professor at the Massachusetts Institute of Technology.

The body can function well for hours or days without food, but it is not natural for the body to be constantly fed. There are evidences, which point that short-term fasting causes autophagy. This is a cellular repair process, where the cells utilize the longstanding protein in your system for energy. This leads to a lot of health benefits that include the protection against Alzheimer's disease, cancer, and aging. Fasting, in general, has good effects on your metabolic health. This is better and healthier than snacking often.

5. Your body will be in starvation mode when you fast.
Adaptive thermogenesis or starvation mode happens when the body reduces the calories it burns. While this may be true, the situation happens no matter what kind of weight loss technique you employ. There are even evidences, which point out that your metabolic rate will increase when you do short-term fasts. The topic was extensively discussed by Martin Berkhan, an expert about IF, on his blog. By engaging in IF, there will be a boost of norepinephrine in your blood. This will trigger fat breakdown and accelerate the metabolic process.

6. The body has a limit in the amount of protein that it can take per meal.
You might have heard from some people that the body can only digest up to 30 grams of protein in every meal. They recommend that you eat after every couple of hours in order to gain muscle. Well, that claim is not supported by any research. The fact is, that the body can take much more than 30 grams of protein, which you can take according to the eating frequency you prefer.

7. You will lose muscle when you follow intermittent fasting.
There is no evidence that proves this claim. Your body will burn some of your muscles as fuel no matter what kind of diet program you follow. It was even concluded in some studies that intermittent fasting may help in maintaining muscle mass while on a diet.

8. Intermittent fasting causes overeating.
Many critics of the diet argue that you won't lose weight when you fast because when you are allowed to eat, there is a tendency that you will eat a lot due to hunger and the feeling of suppression. While it is true that many dieters tend to eat a little more than

usual after fasting, they only do so in order to compensate for the calories that they have lost. For as long as you have your mind set to what you intend to achieve in this kind of diet, you will always remember not to overeat during the hours that you are allowed to break the fast.

Intermittent fasting is effective in helping you lose fat. A 2014 study entitled, *Intermittent Fasting Vs Daily Calorie Restriction for Type 2 Diabetes Prevention* (written by Kristin Hoddy, Adrienne Barnosky, Krista Varady, and Terry G. Unterman), proved that fasting for 3 up to 24 weeks could result to an 8% reduction in body weight and a huge decrease in the fat around the tummy. This is equivalent to 0.55 pounds of weight loss in a week. You can lose a lot more (about 1.65 pounds every week) by engaging in alternate-day fasting.

9. Intermittent fasting is bad for your health.
There are a lot of studies which can prove that the opposite is true. You can gain a lot of health benefits for as long as you fast properly and you do it along with the right diet and exercise. It improves your metabolic health, reduces your susceptibility to heart disease, and enhances your body's sensitivity to insulin.

Your brain will also benefit from the process as it boosts the levels of your BDNF, or the brain-derived neurotrophic factor. As a result, you will have fewer chances of having brain problems and depression. This kind of fasting is good for your health in general. It is also acknowledged as one of the most powerful tools for weight loss.

You are already on the right track by trying to learn more about intermittent fasting. Do not allow these myths to hinder your progress or make you lose sight of the more important benefits of the program.

What are the main perks of engaging in IF?

Intermittent fasting is beneficial in general. It is recommended for people who are intent about losing weight, gaining back their confidence, and getting back in shape and in good health. Many people prefer this kind of diet because it is easy to follow – the rules are lenient, and there are no expensive supplements involved.

Simple and effective – these are the two words that best describe IF. Many people who have gotten over the myths and have tried IF concluded that it carries the following pros:

1. Can you imagine how much money you're going to save because of the meals that you have skipped or the dine-outs that you have refused to be part of? You don't need any fancy meal during your eating windows either. The beauty of it all is that you will benefit from the process despite its simplicity.

2. The diet scheme is flexible. It is up to you to choose the days and time that you are most comfortable with.

3. You don't have to overdo the process if you can't commit to fasting longer than 24 hours. Listen to your body and follow what it says.

4. How does it feel to continually plan what you will eat for a day or for a week? There are times when you will be in the mood to do it, but there will also be times when it would feel dragging. When you are fasting, you'd have plenty of time to plan how you intend to break each fast. The meals are simple and there is no need to fuss over them. It is even better if you can teach yourself to eat the same food each time.

What are the downsides of this kind of diet?
There are some people who find it hard not to eat for long hours. This is a common problem that happens in the beginning.

Consider this as a challenge that you have to get over with. Look forward to the health benefits that you will gain from the process once you have gotten accustomed to the scheme of things.

It is normal to have less energy after trying it for the first time. The idea here is that you must not get discouraged, but do your best to get the hang of things as fast as you can.

Chapter 4 – The Different Methods of Fasting

It is never too late to lose weight. There is no right or wrong time to feel good about yourself. You can do it any time you want. Always remember that whatever kind of diet program you have chosen to follow, the beginning is always the hardest. You simply have to go for it and try out your chosen technique. This will give you ample of time to find out which diet plan won't work and which one suits you best.

IF is as simple as it sounds – you will take in few to no calories for the period of time that you have chosen to fast. The idea here is to choose the type that will suit your lifestyle. Do not force yourself to commit to anything that you cannot religiously follow. This way, there will be higher chances that you will stick to the diet until you have maximized its benefits. The fasting method ought to make your life easier. You have to choose the method that will not make you feel like you are missing out on something.

Intermittent fasting can be categorized into two types – short-term and long-term. Here's a look at the short-term fasting methods:

1. The 12-hour intermittent fasting
This is considered normal and only a little adjustment is needed to follow this kind of fasting every day. It requires three meals each day that you will eat during the hours that are included in your eating window. For example, you have chosen the eating window to fall in between 6AM to 6PM, this means that you will fast and avoid eating anything from 6PM to 6AM. The fast will be broken with a light breakfast.

This kind of fasting is good enough to lose a little weight and avoid obesity. Make sure that you avoid consuming excessive amounts of sugar and unprocessed food.

2. The 16-hour intermittent fasting

This is also done every day. The fasting period will happen for 16 hours, which will leave you with an 8-hour eating window. Many of those who follow the diet choose to skip breakfast each day. The usual time that is allotted for the eating window is from 11AM to 7PM and fasting will begin from 7PM to 11AM.

The method was further developed and later on, popularized by Martin Berkhan, which named it after his website. This is the reason why it is sometimes referred to as the LeanGains method. This is best suited to those who regularly go to the gym and are intent in building muscle and losing fat.

For women, it is recommended to fast for a period of 14 hours per day. Men, on the other hand, should aim for 16 hours. You can eat within the remaining 8 to 10 hours. Make sure that you don't get any calories during the fasting period, but you are allowed to have diet soda, black coffee, sugar-free gum, and calorie-free sweeteners. Most followers of this diet fast through the night, and break it at around six hours upon waking up. You have to make sure that you can stick to the schedule before you commit to it because disrupting the process can affect hormone function.

It is also up to you when to begin the fasting. You should start it depending on the time that you usually work out. What do you eat after the fast? If you will hit the gym after the fast, you have to take in more carbs than fat. On the days that you will take a break from exercising, it is recommended to take in more fat. What will remain the same is your protein consumption. It has to be fairly high each day.

No matter what IF method you have chosen to follow, make sure that you get your calories from whole and unprocessed food. You can also eat a health bar or a protein shake as a meal replacement once in a while, especially if you don't have the time to prepare your own meals.

Many people find it easy to stick to this diet plan since in most days, meal frequency is not relevant. Those who follow it break their feeding time into the three major meals, squeezing them into the periods in which they're allowed to eat.

The downside of the program is that it is stricter with what you can eat because you have to prepare meals that will match the kinds of exercises you often do. It could also be difficult to plan your meals depending on your workout schedule.

3. The Warrior Diet
This is recommended for serious and devoted individuals who can commit and follow the rules. As a warrior or a follower of this diet, you will be required to fast for 20 hours each day and break it by eating a large meal at night. What you eat will contribute to the success of the program so you ought to be careful with your choices. Your body needs essential nutrients, but make sure that you consume foods that are suited for night eating. The 20-hour fast is not that strict. You can actually eat a small serving of fruit or vegetable. In short, the fasting period requires that you under-eat, which is the opposite of what you will do when it is already time to eat. The 4-hour eating period each day can be spent in overeating.

The idea here is that your system will maximize the fight or flight response of your Sympathetic Nervous System during the hours that you are fasting. This will boost your energy, will help you become more alert, and will lead to greater fat burn. The time that you are allowed to eat will maximize the ability of your Parasympathetic Nervous System to help your body recharge and recuperate. This period gives you time to relax and it also aids in digestion.

When you eat at night, your body produces hormones that it utilizes to burn fat during the day. It is important to have a fill of specific food groups during the period that you are allowed to eat. If you are still hungry after you have had a meal that's nutritionally varied (or complete), you can add a little carb into your diet.

Many people like this method because having snacks during the fasting phase is allowed. It makes it easier to adjust to the diet, especially if you're the kind who finds it hard to keep hunger at bay.

The downside of the method is that the types of food that you are allowed to eat after the fast is limited. This will make it hard for you to adjust if you love eating or you always go out with your friends. You always have to remind yourself about what to eat and in what order. The strict guidelines are hard to follow for certain individuals. This is even harder to follow for people who aren't used to eating big meals at night.

If you think that the short-term methods are not helping you attain your weight loss goal, you can try any of the following longer methods of intermittent fasting:

1. Eat Stop Eat
This type is recommended to healthy eaters who want to learn how to practice self-control. This fasting method allows you to eat your favorite foods, but you cannot take as much as you used to.

To get this done, you need to fast for 24 hours once or twice in a week. You cannot eat anything during the fasting period, but it is okay to drink calorie-free fluids. After the 24 hours that you have fasted, you can go back to how you usually eat as if nothing happened. This all boils down to timing. How do you want to end the fast? You can finish it in time for a normal meal and prepare something big and appetizing. You can also end the fast with a light snack in the middle of the afternoon. It all depends on your schedule and preference.

How will it work? The diet will only restrict how often you eat, but it won't limit what you want to eat after the fasting period. The time required for the fasting period is enough to reduce your overall calorie intake. To make the diet work, you have to do regular workout sessions, particularly resistance training. This will trim you down and improve your body composition as well.

The program is actually flexible. You cannot avoid food completely for 24 hours, especially if you are still not used to it. You will give your body the chance to get used to it before you fully commit to this kind of IF. On your first day, it is recommended to listen to your body – find out how far you can go without eating. Go as long as you can without food, but once the craving strikes, go back to eating and stop once your hunger has been satisfied. You can gradually add hours to your fasting period. To make it easier to decide when to begin the fast, choose a date and time when you are not that busy, you won't do too many physical activities, and there are no social gatherings that you are required to attend.

The best thing about this method of IF is that you are not forbidden to eat specific kinds of food. This is easy to follow since you are not required to count calories or restrict what you eat after you have fasted. If you are intent on losing weight, you have to set portions in what you eat. You have to practice eating in moderation. You can also impose the changes gradually in order to give your body enough time to adjust.

What's the downside of the diet? There are certain people who find it hard to go without calories for 24 hours straight. Not a lot of people can easily carry on doing the things that they ought to do without food. Not having anything to eat, especially for an extended period of time, make certain people suffer from side effects that include dizziness, headache, and irritability. It is also tempting to binge on food after fasting for long hours. You have to practice self-control and help yourself to easily adjust to the process. Eventually, you will get used to it and will have lesser episodes of side effects.

2. Alternate Day Fasting
This is suited for those with strict discipline about their diet and those who are intent to achieve their ideal weight. The rules are easy for this IF method – eat a little for a day and eat like how you

normally would the following day. For women, the rule is to stay within 400 calories during the fasting period. For men, the limit is 500 calories.

To make it easier for you to stick to the diet, especially during the fasting period, it is recommended to have meal replacement shakes that you can consume throughout the day rather than splitting your food into small meals. Taking these shakes is only recommended during the first two weeks of the diet program. On the third week, you have to teach your system how to adapt to eating real food during the hours that you need to fast. The following day after the fasting period, you can go back to how you normally eat. After that, you will fast again and then eat normally the following day – continue until it becomes a routine. If you frequent the gym, make sure that you choose a schedule that matches the days when you are allowed to eat normally.

This is ideal for people who are serious about losing weight. By cutting your calorie intake, it is possible to lose up to two and a half pounds every week.

The downside of this program is that you might be tempted to binge on food when you are allowed to eat. If you want to maximize the benefits of the program, you have to impose self-restriction with what you eat and how much, especially during the days that you can eat whatever you want.

3. Fat Loss Forever
This is highly preferred by those who frequent the gym but always look forward to their cheat days. This combines the best parts of many IF methods, plus, you'll get a cheat day every week, which is then followed by 36 hours of fasting. The next day will be split into the different protocols of the various IF methods.

It is normal to get shocked with the 36-hour fasting rule. Many fear that they cannot keep up with it. To make it easier for you, it is recommended to time this rule during the days when you're usually extremely busy. By focusing on how to be productive and how to finish the tasks that you have already started, you can get your mind off from hunger and your cravings.

This method requires that you sign up for a program and follow a 7-day plan. The plan will be based on your age, weight, and physical activities. A timetable will be designed depending on your workload and how much weight you intend to lose.

The downside of the program is that the cheat days can actually backfire on you. It is important to eat in moderation even when it is your cheat day. If you will not impose self-restriction, it might be hard for you to go back to eating less or eating nothing at all.

4. The 24-hour intermittent fasting

This has many similarities to the Warrior method of fasting. It also allows a 4-hour eating window. Technically, fasting will last for 20 hours. You can choose the fasting time depending on which suits you the best. Some people do it from breakfast to breakfast, while others prefer fasting from dinner to dinner. It means that you will have one meal each day.

This is beneficial and healthier, especially to people who are taking medications. They can take their meds after they have eaten during the allotted period. This method of fasting is relatively easy to adopt. You can, for example, take your one meal in time for dinner, which you can have with your family. No one will notice that you have skipped breakfast and lunch. This will also work if you are an extremely busy person. You can begin the day with a cup of coffee, get busy with work, and then recharge when you get home in time for dinner.

Allow Your Body to Adjust
No matter what method you have chosen to follow, it will not be easy to get adjusted to the process. It is important to start slow

and allow your body to get used to the changes before you fully commit to that plan.

Fasting is not suited for everyone. You have to tell your doctor about it if you are suffering from any medical condition or if you are undergoing special diet programs. You must also plan ahead before you commit to the process. Make sure that you are ready in all aspects, especially with the food that you ought to consume after the fasting phase.

Chapter 5 – Essential Tips to Make the Diet Work

Here are some tips that will make it easier for you to begin with any IF method and stick with it:

1. Keep yourself hydrated by drinking plenty of water. This will make you feel full even during your fasting hours. It will make it easier for you to stick to your diet program. Begin your day by drinking water first thing upon waking up. You may have noticed that you typically feel hungry in the morning. The reason for this is the lack of water intake while you were sleeping for 8 hours or so. For weight loss purposes, the ideal amount of water that you ought to consume upon waking up is at least half liter. For men, it's important to drink up to 4 liters of water daily. For women, 2 liters is enough.

2. When planning for your fasting schedule, make sure that most of the time that you will spend fasting will be done at night while you sleep. This will make it easier for you to keep your mind away from food, avoid temptations, and lessen your cravings.

3. It is better to start fasting when you are busy. This will keep your mind away from eating because you will be more focused on finishing your tasks and in keeping yourself busy with the things that you ought to finish. Many people are more compelled to give their best at work when they have not eaten. This is something that you have to learn as you go on with your diet.

Make a list of what you need to accomplish for each day. Finish all your routines upon waking up and get started on your tasks. This way, you can get many things done even before you are reminded of hunger.

4. Never feel like you are depriving yourself of food simply because you are fasting. You have to think of it as a break period from eating. Do not spend the fasting period thinking about what to eat

when it's time to break the fast. Fill your mind with thoughts other than food. Consider this your break time not only from eating, but also in thinking about food.

5. Make sure that you don't forget to exercise. Follow exercise programs that will suit your lifestyle and the method of IF that you are following. Here's something to keep in mind though – there are certain exercises, such as cardio, which can trigger hunger. If you feel the same way, go ahead and look for other exercises that you can do to keep your body fit and to help in making you forget about your hunger.

6. Take branched-chain amino acids or BCAAs. There are evidences which can prove that taking them while you are on a diet can speed up the fat loss. The term refers to three essential amino acids – valine, leucine and isoleucine, which all come with a special branched structure. They comprise a third of your skeletal muscle. It is ideal to consume BCAA when you are under a low-calorie diet. This will speed up the loss of your visceral fat.

It is vital to take BCAAs when you are constantly training because they can help reduce muscle breakdown. The ideal consumption is around 12 grams each day. The result is maximized fat loss, leaner muscles, and greater ease in maintaining your ideal weight and shape.

7. Keep stock cubes handy. If you feel like you can't control your hunger anymore, you can always drink a stock cube soup. A quarter of the soup contains around 3 calories. You can cut it in half if you want. Many dieters take it before going to bed, so that they will find it easier to sleep because their mind won't end up focusing on hunger.

8. Avoid overeating by going for the same foods as much as you can. This will kill the excitement of looking forward to what you can have during the hours of your eating window.

9. It is up to you whether or not you will tell other people that you are fasting. If it is going to help and you are certain that you will get the needed support, then go ahead and share with them what you're trying to do. If you think that people will only question your decisions and mock you for what you are doing, then it is best to keep it a secret. You can choose the right people to share the information with. You might need them to boost your spirits whenever you feel low or you're on the verge of giving up.

10. You can drink coffee or tea whenever you feel like it during the day. Caffeine is known as a natural appetite suppressant. Make sure that you don't drink too much, or else, you might feel anxious. Well, aside from that, be sure not to drink it several hours before bedtime.

11. Never give up too soon. It is true that you have to find the right method of IF that will work for you. This can only be done through trial and error. The ideal trial period is at least three weeks. This will give you enough time to adjust and monitor if your body is going through any change. If nothing is happening or you are not really getting used to the scheme of things, then it is best to move on and try another IF method. Just keep on doing it until you have found the best method that will give you the most health benefits.

Chapter 6 – Frequently Asked Questions about Intermittent Fasting

To make it easier for you to understand and remember the important points about the process, here are the frequently asked question about it, with the corresponding answers:

1. Can everybody do intermittent fasting?
Definitely not. Similar to other kinds of diet programs, IF is not suitable for everybody. The following are not suited to undergo any IF method:

- People who are under 18 years of age
- Pregnant women and breastfeeding mothers
- Those who have recently undergone surgery
- Those who are suffering from any eating disorder
- People who are malnourished or underweight
- Those who have or are recuperating from fever
- People suffering from or have a history of serious mental health concerns
- Diabetics, especially the ones taking prescription medications

It is also not recommended for children and teens. Their bodies will undergo a lot of natural changes, so it is best that they wait until they become adults before trying IF or any other kind of diet programs. Healthy adults can undergo IF, but old people who are frail and often get sick must stay away from the process and similar techniques.

2. Can someone who doesn't have any weight problem follow intermittent fasting?
IF has many benefits aside from weight loss. The only way to determine if this is going to be beneficial to your health is to choose a method that suits you best and try it firsthand. Even

though your weight is normal, your cells will still benefit from the duration that you will allot to fasting because it boosts the maintenance and repair processes.

Aside from addressing health concerns, fasting has been advocated by many religious groups and is being followed as part of rituals and devotion. Even for those not into religion, fasting could be an excellent means of developing self-control.

3. How do you begin doing IF?
Adjusting may be the hardest part for a lot of individuals who are trying it out for the first time. You have to find ways to make it easier to begin, commit, and learn how to make it part of your lifestyle. Make sure that you choose a starting day when there is less temptation to eat. You can start the diet at the time when you are extremely busy that you'd barely think about food. You have to plan ahead and know beforehand what you will eat during the hours that you are allowed to.

4. Is it more effective to fast for consecutive or non-consecutive days?
Actually, it doesn't matter, for as long as you are comfortable doing the fast on the days that you have chosen to do it. There are some dieters, for example, who fast for two consecutive days, while others do it at the beginning and the middle of the week.

5. How long does a fast day last?
A day that you will spend fasting should actually last for 36 hours. For example, you had your last full meal on Sunday at 7PM. You will then have your fast day on Monday, which will last until 7AM on Tuesday. This is an ideal scenario since you had your last meal at dinnertime and your next meal after the fast will be in the morning. This is the reason why it is important to plan ahead when it comes to the time you'll begin and end each fast day.

6. What can be eaten during the hours that it is allowed to eat, and how often should one eat?
The number of times that you can eat per day depends on the method of fasting that you have chosen to follow. It can be one big meal at lunch, several small meals spread throughout the day, two major meals each day, and so on. You have to read how each method is done so that you can wisely choose the type that you can stick to and be comfortable with. There is no best method when it comes to this kind of diet. It varies among individuals, depending on activity level and kind of lifestyle.

Make sure that you take in sufficient nutrients, such as protein and fiber, which you can get from various food sources (including meat, veggies, and fish). There are also foods that you need to avoid during your fast days, specifically the kinds that are loaded with refined carbs and sugar. If you are intent on losing weight, then you must have prepared to drop the delicacies that you used to enjoy, such as ice cream, sweet pastries, rice, potatoes, and pasta.

You can still have some snacks, but this is not the right time to be picky. You can eat something raw to feed your hunger, such as slices of carrots, apple with skin, celery sticks, or a handful of almonds. The list may not sound as appetizing as the foods that you ought to avoid, but you will eventually get used to it. You simply have to think about the benefits of the process all the time, so that you will find it easier to commit.

For the drinks, you have to consume a lot of water in order to stay hydrated even while fasting. You can drink anything that has little or no calories, such as coffee or tea. If you want to drink any alcoholic beverage, it is better that you postpone it until your fast day is over. You must not consume too much alcohol because it's actually loaded with calories, meaning it can cause a spike in your insulin levels.

7. Are there easy ways to count calories when you fast?
To make it easier for you to plan meals with the right amount of calories, it is recommended to follow recipes with caloric values listed. You can also use free calorie counters that can be found on many websites. You will eventually get the hang of things, and you'll be able to effortlessly determine the amount of calories based on the ingredients and the quantity that you are allowed to consume.

8. Can you fast if you are not feeling well?
It depends on the cause of your sickness, but it is actually best to skip fasting when you are unwell. You need all the nutrients that you can get when you are sick in order to help yourself get better at a faster rate. You might get worse if you are not going to eat. Fasting will also cause stress. This is your body's natural response in order to prompt the repair process. While it helps during the fast days, it will do the opposite if you're sick.

9. Is it allowed to exercise when you are fasting?
Yes, but you must not overdo it and you have to listen to your body when it is time to stop. As revealed in several studies, those who exercise while fasting burn more fat. Other studies suggest that men who work out before having their breakfast was able to burn more fat than those who only exercised after the fast day. Aside from burning fat, exercising can give you a good distraction when your mind is starting to crave for food.

10. What if the method that you have chosen isn't helping you lose weight?
This is where the flexibility of the process comes in. Even when you have already started with a method, you can adjust it or choose to follow a different method if it is not helping you in attaining your goal. For one, you can add another fast day and make it, for example, 4:3. If you have already reached a plateau with the said method, you can try doing the Alternate Day Fasting or ADF.

It is more ideal that you think more about losing fat than obsessing about your weight. Instead of constantly checking how much you weigh, it is better if you will monitor the changes in your measurements, especially around the gut area, as you continue to fast.

When you are not fasting, you have to be always on a lookout with regards to the calorie content of the food and drinks you consume. Make sure that you stay away from anything that contains too many calories and sugar. It is also recommended to keep on moving a lot. It is ideal to do around 10,000 steps each day. You can use a pedometer to make it easier for you to monitor your steps. The exercise is something that you can adopt even after you have stopped fasting or have chosen to try another diet technique.

11. How often should one's weight be monitored and what is the best way to get your body's measurement?
You can get your weight at the end of each week to learn about your progress. Again, it is more important to monitor fat loss, especially around the waist area, than to obsess about your weight. To effectively measure your waist, stand with your feet apart. Breathe like you normally would and begin measuring directly against the skin, but make sure that the tape measure is not compressing your skin even a bit. The measurement must start in the middle point of the lowest rib to the top of the hip bone, almost touching your belly button.

12. Does this kind of diet come with side effects?
Similar to other diet techniques, the first side effect of this program is hunger. This is normal in the beginning while you are still giving your body time to adjust to the changes. This might be more difficult at night, especially when you are not used to sleeping on an empty stomach.

In this case, you can have a late night snack to satiate the craving. It is not likely that you'd suffer from constipation and headaches, but if you experience them as side effects, this means that there is something wrong with what you are doing.

You have to drink more water during the day in order to prevent these. There are also studies which point out that a person is likely experience the side effects that he's expecting to experience even before starting the program. In this case, it is best that you only have positive expectations when you decide to commit to the program.

Fat is energy dense. This is the reason why it takes a long time to burn, especially as you age. There will really come a time when you would need the help of diet programs and learning how to use readily-available ingredients, such as coconut oil, to speed up the process. It is important to remember that you cannot overcompensate for the nutrients of which you have deprived yourself during your fast days.

It's normal to feel shaky after fasting for several hours. There are certain people who feel like they would faint after a couple of days without food. You can counter the feeling because it's all in the mind, unless you are diabetic. For healthy individuals, it is only natural for the body to maintain proper blood sugar levels and it will keep on doing so after fasting for several days.

13. How hungry can you get?
There will be times when you will be reminded of hunger, but the moments will pass. You can help yourself get through the phase by drinking a calorie-free drink, going for a walk, or by doing anything that could provide the needed distraction.

The belief that you will be in starvation mode when you fast is only a myth. The body naturally increases your metabolic rate when your calorie intake is reduced.

14. Does fasting affect gout?
It is not likely to happen with intermittent fasting. IF can help in reducing your inflammation, which can get worse if you suffer from dehydration. Make sure that you drink lots of fluids throughout the day while you are fasting. To lessen your risk of

gout in general, consume less foods that are rich in purine, such as sardines, cauliflower, alcohol, oatmeal, liver, and lentils.

15. Is it safe to fast after undergoing an operation?
It is best not to force your body to fast a few weeks after a minor operation and around two months after undergoing a major operation. It is better if you will keep a high protein diet while recuperating in order to boost the healing process.

16. How do you monitor the changes when undergoing this kind of fasting?
Make sure that you monitor your weight and measure the changes in your waist, hips, and chest. In order to ensure that your health is okay, it is also recommended to keep track of your resting pulse rate. You can use certain devices at home in order to monitor your blood pressure, fasting glucose, and cholesterol. If you can't do it on your own, ask your doctor about it or go to a licensed clinic and get the tests done.

17. How can it be easy to maintain the weight that was lost after reaching the target?
It is best to fast a day each week after you have reached your target. Keep a calorie-restricted diet in order to keep and maintain what you have already started.

Again and again, you will hear people telling you how important it is to make fasting a way of life. Through time, you will discover how to tweak the diet in order to make it more suitable to the kind of lifestyle that you are leading. There will also come a time when you will learn how to control your cravings and know the kinds of foods that are beneficial to your overall health. You have to make the diet work for you by making it flexible. You have the freedom when to begin and end each fast. It should never inhibit with your daily routine.

Chapter 7 – Foods for Weight Loss

How do you break the fast? What are the ingredients that you need to stock up on? Here are some of the best ingredients for weight loss:

Coconut oil
Coconut oil is one ingredient that must be part of any kind of low-carb diet. This oil will help you in achieving two of the most important goals of IF – losing weight and boosting energy. What's so special about this oil and how can you use it?

- Coconut oil enhances your system's ability to digest food, speeding up the process of burning body fat. As a result, it will be easier for your body to absorb the nutrients from the food that you eat.

- It gives you more energy. This is due to its important component, which is the medium-chain triglyceride (MCT) lauric acid.

- Daily intake of coconut oil can suppress your hunger and food cravings. If you find it hard to consume the oil on its own, you can mix this with your drinks or add it to your food.

- Taking it daily can make your digestive tract healthier and more capable of absorbing fat-soluble vitamins.

- The oil helps in balancing your hormones. This will result to better digestion and improved mood, metabolism, and sex drive. The oil makes it easier for your system to burn stored fats, specifically in the problem areas, such as the tummy, waist, and thighs.

- It regulates your blood sugar levels. The oil acts on the food that you take, so your body uses a little of its digestive enzymes. Your pancreas is not overworked, and that is why it is able to produce insulin without any hassle. The oil, being a saturated fat, gets mixed with insulin upon digestion. In effect, your body gets a sufficient supply of glucose or blood sugar.

Coconut oil is now being tagged as the most weight-loss-friendly fat in the world because of its composition and health benefits. Despite this, you must bear in mind that this is still oil and it has a high calorie content. Make sure that you do not go beyond the recommended daily limit, which is three tablespoons.

You can try the following ways of including this oil into your diet in order to get your needed energy boost:

- Use the oil in preparing and cooking healthy dishes, such as salad, curry, and stir-fried or sautéed vegetables.

- Take it like how you would take a vitamin pill. Limit your daily intake to two to three tablespoons each day, especially when you are already old. Remember that the oil has energy boosting effects, so do not take this before you sleep. This will make you toss and turn all night.

- Drink coconut milk because it still contains the oil that you need. You can also try eating coconut meat.

- You can eat raw coconut, but make sure that it is mature, has a brown color, and a hard shell. This is the type of coconut where the healthy oil is obtained from.

Cutting Your Carb Intake
This is the essence of your diet. Fasting will not work if you will not cut your carb intake. Doing so will lead to a significant reduction of your hunger. Make this part of your lifestyle along with fasting, and you will automatically lose weight without the need to count calories. This is also beneficial to your health and it isn't complicated at all.

Here's a list of low-carb foods that you can mix and match or prepare in a variety of ways:

1. Eggs. This is considered among the most nutritious foods. You can use it in many dishes and it can be prepared by itself in a lot of ways. The carb content of an egg is almost zero, yet it is loaded with nutrients and healthy compounds that are good for the eye and brain.

2. Fish and seafood. They are rich in omega-3 fatty acids, vitamin B12, and iodine. Most of them have a little or no carbs at all. Here are a few good examples:

- Salmon. It contains zero carbs, but is loaded with vitamin D3, B12, and iodine. This fatty fish has a good dose of omega-3 fatty acids that are good for the heart.
- Sardines. They also contain zero carbs and are among the most nutrient-dense foods. They contain almost all kinds of nutrients that your body needs and the best thing about them is that you can eat them whole.

- Trout. This is another kind of fatty fish that is rich in omega-3 fatty acids. It also contains zero carbs.
- Shellfish. They contain small amounts of carbs, about 5 grams for every 100 grams. They are among the most nutritious foods and are loaded with nutrients.
- Other good examples include herring, haddock, tuna, shrimp, catfish, lobster, cod, and halibut.

3. Meats. All kinds of meat contain little or zero carbs.

- Lamb. This meat is loaded with nutrients, such as vitamin B12 and iron. It also contains high levels of a healthy fatty acid called conjugated linoleic acid or CLA.
- Beef. It is tasty and nutritious. It can be served in many ways and you can get this meat in various forms, such as hamburger, ribeye steak, or ground.
- Chicken. For the kind of diet that you have, it is recommended to get the fattier cuts, such as the thighs and wings.
- Pork. This is nutritious and delicious. You can also include bacon in your food list, but make sure that you only take it in moderation. However, avoid bacon that has lots of preservatives and is cured in sugar.
- Other meats you could try include venison, turkey, bison, and veal.

4. Vegetables

This diet requires that you eat your greens, especially the cruciferous and leafy kinds. Stay away from starchy root veggies that are high in carbs, such as sweet potatoes and potatoes.

- Tomatoes. These are considered fruits or berries, but are mostly eaten as veggies. They contain healthy nutrients, such as potassium and vitamin C.
- Broccoli. This is rich in fiber, vitamins K and C, and other cancer-fighting compounds. It's tasty and can be eaten raw or cooked.
- Brussels Sprouts. They have the same levels of nutrients as broccoli and can be served in a variety of ways.
- Cauliflower. This is another versatile vegetable. It also contains high levels of folate, vitamin K, and vitamin C.
- Onions. They are tasty and give a strong flavor to your dishes. Aside from that, they're rich in anti-inflammatory compounds, fiber, and antioxidants.
- Kale. This healthy vegetable contains high amounts of carotene antioxidants, vitamin C, vitamin K, and fiber.
- Cucumber. It has a mild flavor because it mostly contains water (but it does have a little amount of vitamin K).
- Eggplant. This is also a fruit that is mostly eaten as a vegetable. It is high in fiber and can be enjoyed in many ways.
- Asparagus. This delicious vegetable has a good dose of protein, and nutrients, such as vitamin C, fiber, folate, antioxidants, and vitamin K.
- Mushrooms. They contain high amounts of vitamin B and potassium.
- Bell Peppers. These are known for their satisfying and distinct flavor, and they contain high levels of carotene antioxidants, fiber, and vitamin C.

- Green beans. These legumes are loaded with nutrients, including protein, magnesium, fiber, vitamin K, potassium, and vitamin C.
- For greater variety, you may try these other veggies – Swiss chard, spinach, cabbage, celery, and zucchini.

5. Fruits and berries

Because they contain more carbs than veggies, it is important to limit your intake of fruits to a couple of pieces each day. There is an exception to the rule though. There are fatty fruits (such as olives and avocado) and berries with low sugar content (like strawberries), which you can indulge on.

- Avocado. It is a unique fruit because it contains a good dose of healthy fats and only a little amount of carbs. This is also rich in potassium, fiber, and other healthy nutrients.
- Olives. This high-fat fruit is delicious and nutritious. It contains healthy nutrients, such as copper, iron, and vitamin E.
- Strawberries. They are among the most-nutrient dense fruits. Despite containing minimal carbs, they're rich in manganese, antioxidants, and vitamin C.
- Apricots. Aside from being delicious, they are loaded with potassium and vitamin C. Also, they're not loaded with carbohydrates.
- Grapefruit. This citrus fruit is rich in carotene antioxidants and vitamin C.
- Raspberries, oranges, lemons, mulberries, and kiwi are other excellent choices.

6. Fats and oils

There are many fats and oils that you can include in your diet, but avoid refined vegetable oils that can be unhealthy when taken in excess. These unhealthy oils include corn oil and soybean oil, and the healthy and low-carb types include the following:

- Extra virgin olive oil. It is considered the healthiest fat and is rich in anti-inflammatory elements and antioxidants. It's good for your cardiovascular health and can be served as part of many dishes, including the heart-healthy meals of a Mediterranean diet.
- Butter. It has zero carb content and contains high doses of nutrients. It is recommended to choose the grass-fed type of butter.
- Other examples of fats and oils include lard, tallow, and avocado oil.

7. Nuts and seeds

Nuts can be eaten as snacks, while seeds are typically incorporated into recipes, such as salads. They are both staples of low-carb diets because they are rich in micronutrients, fat, protein, and fiber.

- Almonds. These nuts are filling, crunchy, and tasty. They are also rich in magnesium, Vitamin E, and fiber.
- Peanuts. They are loaded with vitamin E, fiber, magnesium, and other vitamins and minerals.
- Walnuts. They are delicious and contain high levels of the omega-3 fatty acid ALA.
- Chia seeds. This is included in the list of the most popular health foods in the world. They are loaded with dietary fiber and other essential nutrients. The seeds can be added to various low-carb recipes.

- You may also enjoy coconuts, macadamia nuts, flax seeds, hazelnuts, pumpkin seeds, sunflower seeds, cashews, and pistachios.

8. Beverages. You can have any sugar-free drink. Do make sure to avoid fruit juices because they are loaded with carbs and sugar.

- Water
- Tea. Different kinds of tea offer numerous health benefits.
- Coffee. It is rich in antioxidants and helps in reducing your risk of certain diseases, such as Parkinson's, Alzheimer's and type 2 diabetes. This is best taken as black, but to add variation, you can also take it with heavy cream or full-fat milk.
- Carbonated water/Club soda. This is only water with carbon monoxide. Choose the kind without added sugars.

9. Condiments and herbs. They add flavor to your dishes and they contain low amounts of carbs, but are rich in nutrients.

- Salt
- Pepper
- Cinnamon
- Oregano
- Garlic
- Mustard

10. Dark chocolate. Who says that you can't have a treat while on a low-carb diet? Just make sure that you buy real dark choco that's at least 80 percent cocoa. It is known for numerous health benefits that include lower blood pressure, decreased susceptibility to heart ailments, and healthier brain function.

11. Dairy products

Full-fat dairy is suitable for your diet, but make sure that you avoid the kinds with added sugar.

- Heavy cream. It is high in fat, but low in carbs and protein. You can take it with your coffee or with a bowl of fruits or berries.
- Cheese. It is tasty and can be used in many recipes or eaten as it is. Don't forget that it's nutritious as well. One slice of cheese contains the same amount of nutrients as a glass of milk.
- Greek yogurt. This is also called strained yogurt, which is thicker than the regular kinds of yogurt. It is rich in protein and other nutrients, but has low carb content. It also has a distinct flavor that's not ideal for snacking, so try to add it to your dishes instead.
- Full-fat yogurt. This is as nutritious as whole milk, but has added nutrients. Of course, it contains healthy probiotics. These gut microbes allow you to maximize the nutrients you get from food, and protect you from illnesses caused by the proliferation of bad bacteria.

Conclusion

I hope this book was able to help you to learn more about intermittent fasting. The details are meant to inspire you to take advantage of its benefits and start adapting the process into your lifestyle. It's now time to prepare yourself – choose a date and plan your activities to begin fasting.

As you engage in your weight loss endeavor though, be sure to note any changes in your body. While it's important to track the pounds you shed, you shouldn't overlook anything that could be a bad sign. Again, it's recommended to do IF with the guidance of a dietitian or a physician.

Thank you again for purchasing this book!

Can I Ask for a HUGE Favor?

If you enjoyed this book, found it useful or otherwise then I'd really appreciate it if you would post a short review on Amazon. I do read all the reviews personally so that I can continually write what people are wanting and help them achieve success with their fitness goals.

Thanks for your support!

Other Titles by Steve Blum

Atkins Diet: Break Out from the Fat Prison for Good

Ketosis Diet: 30 Day Plan for Optimal, Super-Effective Fat Loss with Ketogenic Diet

Made in the USA
Lexington, KY
19 October 2017